THE *CELLULITE* BREAKTHROUGH

5 STEPS TO ENDING CELLULITE FOREVER

Maggie Greenwood-Robinson, *Ph.D.*

D1560205

A Dell Book

Published by
Dell Publishing
a division of
Random House, Inc.
1540 Broadway
New York, New York 10036

Cover photo courtesy of PNI.

Dell books may be purchased for business or promotional use or for special sales. For information please write to: Special Markets Department, Random House, Inc., New York, NY 10036.

Dell® is a registered trademark of Random House, Inc., and the colophon is a trademark of Random House, Inc.

ISBN: 0-440-23615-0

Printed in the United States of America

Published simultaneously in Canada

May 2000

10 9 8 7 6 5 4 3 2 1

OPM

To John Parrillo
for his lasting contributions to health and fitness

ACKNOWLEDGMENTS

I gratefully thank the following people for their work and contributions to this book: my agent, Madeleine Morel, 2M Communications, Ltd.; Maggie Crawford and the staff at The Bantam Dell Publishing Group; Margie D. Adelman of the Transmedia Group; Chris Eberhard for his photography; Bob Bruce for his artwork; Jeff Wade of the Edge Health & Fitness Center in Newburgh, Indiana, for allowing me to his facility for photography; and my husband Jeff, for love and patience during the research and writing of this book.

CONTENTS

PART V: SUPPORTIVE TREATMENTS

INTRODUCTION

Hear the word "cellulite," and you immediately visualize lumpy-looking, puckered skin. Chances are, you have it. Now the question is: Can you get rid of it?

Women ask me this all the time. They've heard that you can't, that it's hopeless to try. Not true! There is much you can do to eliminate cellulite, or at least minimize it. All it takes is a willingness to try and some commitment to keep at it.

I am forty-seven years old. I have many of the factors that predispose a woman to developing cellulite: body shape, age, a tendency to put on weight, struggles with water retention, relatives who have cellulite, and a family history of varicose veins and lax, loose skin. Most of the cellulite-developing cards have been stacked against me!

Yet I have very minimal cellulite. The reason is that for years I have followed a nutritious diet and have regularly taken supplements such as *Gingko biloba,* vitamin C, agents called OPCs, and other nutrients that have recently been proven to combat cellulite. I have strength-trained for more than twenty years and have practiced a specialized form of anticellulite stretching that I learned from its developer. I also do aerobics to burn body fat and practice ballet to lengthen my muscles and stay flexible. Taken together, these habits have kept my body *cellulite resistant*.

Becoming cellulite resistant is largely a matter of lifestyle. That's incredibly good news! By changing your lifestyle, you can make your body cellulite resistant too. And you can do it *naturally*.

"Naturally" is the operative word in treating and eliminating cellulite. Don't think for one moment that you can have it vacuumed out by liposuction, either. Liposuction isn't even designed to remove cellulite. It has an entirely different purpose. In fact, when a plastic surgeon performs liposuction, he or she purposely bypasses cellulite-affected skin to go after another type of fat, located in the deep layers of skin.

The only methods that really work against cellulite are natural ones—diet, supplementation, special exercises, and supportive treatments that minimize its appearance. How do I know they work? Partly because of my own experience. But more important, because of the scientific proof that has been accumulating on the prevention and treatment of cellulite through natural therapies.

Cellulite is no longer a silly problem being pooh-poohed by the medical establishment. It is now being taken seriously by physicians, medical researchers, and other health care professionals. Doctors are endorsing the research behind anticellulite supplements. Dermatologists are scientifically investigating cellulite as a bona fide skin problem. Plastic surgeons are even beginning to treat it with natural therapies.

Thus, much of the information in this book is cutting-edge, thanks to an ever-expanding base of research on cellulite and its treatment. I have organized this book into five parts: a primer on cellulite, anticellulite supplements, anticellulite nutrition, anticellulite exercise, and supportive treatments. Within each part are chapters that cover specific aspects of cellulite treatment and prevention.

I have also included a 30-Day Anticellulite Diet, found in

chapter 8. It contains satisfying 1000-to-1400-calorie-a-day meal plans that tell you exactly what to eat each day of the week for thirty days. You don't have to worry about the nutrition, either. All the nutrients you need for vitality and good health are built right into the plan. You can adapt these menus to match your own food preferences too.

There is also an easy-to-follow Anticellulite Workout, located in chapter 12. It doesn't take much time to perform, plus you can do it in the convenience of your own home, if you wish.

While it's best to read this book sequentially—that is, from cover to cover—you can also skip around and quickly locate the information you need. My hope is that you'll keep this book handy, as a guide and a motivator. It has been my goal to make the information easy to understand, easy to find, and easy to refer to.

Using this recently discovered, practical information, you'll learn how to make your body cellulite resistant too—and feel great about yourself at the same time.

Maggie Greenwood-Robinson, Ph.D.

CHAPTER 1

Toward a Cellulite-Resistant Body

You slowly turn your back to the mirror. There it is. That dreaded puckered skin on the back of your hips, thighs, and buttocks.

You know it when you see it: cellulite.

Cellulite gives your outer skin an orange peel or cottage-cheesy appearance. It has also been described as spongy, puckered, or indented like a mattress.

No one wants cellulite, yet most of us have it—eight out of every ten women, to be exact.

What is this imperfection called cellulite—and can anything be done about it?

Understanding Cellulite

Cellulite is not a disease or a medical problem, but rather a recognized cosmetic condition related to the underlying structure of the skin. It is characterized by a lax, dimpled skin surface covering the thighs, buttocks, and hips. Doctors and medical researchers who study cellulite have drawn numerous conclusions about it. Cellulite:

- begins to develop during or after puberty.
- varies in severity from person to person.
- is progressive, if interventional treatments are not pursued.
- is found in women of all races.
- is not necessarily related to being overweight, although excess weight worsens the condition.
- is found in slender women too.
- rarely appears in men, regardless of their weight, except in men who are deficient in certain hormones called androgens.
- has numerous causes.
- is not painful.
- can be successfully treated with natural methods.

A misconception exists that cellulite is a type of body fat. In fact, cellulite is a condition in which the outer layer of skin turns dimpled in appearance as a result of structural changes taking place beneath the skin's surface. To help you better understand cellulite, let's take a close look at the underlying structure of your skin and the anatomy of cellulite.

The Structure of Skin

The skin is the largest organ of the body, covering approximately two square yards if you stretched it out like a tablecloth. Anatomically, it is made up of two layers—the epidermis and the dermis. The epidermis is the visible top layer. Its outermost surface is made up of dead skin cells; living skin cells lie just underneath.

The dermis, situated below the epidermis, makes up the bulk of your skin—about 90 percent. The dermis provides strength and gives elasticity to your skin. It is composed of elastic yellow fibers called elastin, and strong white fibers known as collagen.

Collagen deserves some explanation because of the important role it plays in skin and tissue firmness. It is the most abundant protein in the body and makes up about 6 percent of our weight. Structurally, each collagen fiber is twisted together like a rope. Collagen is very strong tissue, with enough toughness and resiliency to spring back after being pulled or compressed.

Although distributed mostly in the connective tissue, collagen also gives shape to vital organs. It forms a fine scaffolding for organ cells and blood vessels so that they can arrange themselves into their characteristic shapes. Collagen literally binds our bodies together.

Along with collagen fibers, there are blood vessels, muscle cells, nerves, lymph vessels, hair follicles, and glands interspersed throughout the dermis too.

As you get older, the dermis becomes thinner and less elastic—the result of a declining number of "mother cells" in the skin. Technically referred to as fibroblasts, mother cells give birth to new collagen and elastin. But with their age-related decline, collagen and elastin production slows down, and skin elasticity decreases.

Beneath the dermis is the subcutaneous fat layer, which also contains a network of blood vessels, lymph vessels, and nerves.

Most of the fat in the subcutaneous layer is referred to as storage fat. It is the type we are always trying to get rid of. Although most storage fat is found in the subcutaneous fat layer, some storage fat pads organs for protection.

There is also a type of fat called essential fat. It is the structural constituent of vital body parts such as the brain, nerve tissue, bone marrow, heart, and cell membranes. Women have about 12 to 15 percent essential fat. Overall, you have about 20 billion to 30 billion fat cells in your body—enough fat to fuel a forty-day fast.

Subcutaneous fat is composed of two layers separated by a sheet of connective tissue known as the fascia. The deeper of the two layers is technically referred to as localized fat deposits (LFDs). LFDs are the primary fat targeted for removal in the surgical procedure known as liposuction. (See Appendix A for more information on liposuction.) The fat cells found in LFDs enlarge faster than other fat cells in the body and are very resistant to dieting. The "saddlebags" on some women's thighs are aggregates of LFDs.

The Anatomy of Cellulite

Cellulite is located in the uppermost layer of subcutaneous fat. This layer is structurally compartmentalized in tiny upright chambers arched like church windows. These chambers are encircled and separated by vertical bands of connective tissue called septa. They are anchored to the dermis above and the fascia below. This architecture resembles a honeycomb.

In women, the fat chambers tend to be large and irregularly shaped. By contrast, in men these chambers are smaller and neatly structured in uniform, polygon-shaped units.

The fat cells inside these chambers can increase up to three hundred times their original size. When this occurs, too much fat becomes crammed inside these chambers. The overstuffed chambers make the skin jut out, creating that all-too-familiar, quiltlike appearance over the outer surface of your hips, thighs, and buttocks.

Compounding the problem are structural weaknesses involving the septa, the connective tissue. With age and other factors, the septa shrinks and thickens, pulling the skin downward—much like the stitching that holds mattress tucks down. This causes the characteristic indentations in the outer skin. The net effect of overstuffed fat chambers and shortened septa is cellulite.

What Actually Triggers Cellulite?

Recent scientific evidence points to multiple reasons for changes in skin and fat architecture that lead to cellulite. This is good news, because identified causes lead to effective treatments. Here's what we know about the mechanisms that contribute to the formation of cellulite, and aggravate its appearance.

INCREASED COLLAGEN BREAKDOWN

Although it is very strong, collagen can be broken down by enzymes that occur naturally in the skin—a reaction triggered by the female hormone estrogen (see below). Collagen breakdown produces some corresponding symptoms that lead to cellulite: water retention, swelling, and pressure on the fat chambers. Consequently, fat extrudes, or bulges, from its chambers, creating the characteristic dimpled appearance of cellulite.

HORMONES

The female hormone estrogen plays a role in the development of cellulite. Estrogen is the collective name for a trio of female hormones: estradiol, secreted from the ovaries during reproductive years; estriol, produced by the placenta during pregnancy; and estrone, secreted by the ovaries and adrenal glands and found in women after menopause.

These naturally occurring estrogens are responsible for developing the female sex characteristics, regulating the menstrual cycle, and maintaining normal cholesterol levels.

Among its many other duties, estrogen causes your body to store excess fat—usually on your thighs, hips, and buttocks. This is partly nature's doing. You need that fat for menstruation, pregnancy, and lactation. It's only during lactation that the body willingly gives up fat cells in these regions, and it does this to support the energy needs of the nursing baby. In any event, cellulite can worsen in some women when estrogen levels spike upward—during puberty, adolescence, and pregnancy.

Estrogen is also responsible for altering the underlying architecture of your skin, giving the fat chambers and septa the irregular pattern that is characteristic of a woman's anatomy. This change occurs at puberty.

In addition, estrogen can act on enzymes to break down collagen and elastin, a protein similar to collagen that gives skin its elasticity. It is well known that estrogen acts in this manner, since the breakdown of collagen is necessary to relax the cervix just prior to childbirth. The breakdown of collagen and elastin in the hips, thighs, and buttocks, however, increases the severity of cellulite.

During menopause—which typically occurs between ages forty-five and fifty-five—your body starts producing less estrogen. Estrogen replacement therapy is often recommended for preventing diseases such as osteoporosis and for generally maintaining good health beyond menopause. In fact, studies show that women who take estrogen for up to ten years have a 37 percent lower risk of premature death.

Some medical experts feel that estrogen replacement therapy can promote cellulite formation and make it difficult to treat. If you are considering estrogen replacement therapy, you must weigh these issues and discuss them with your physician. At this stage in your life, the preservation of overall health may be more important than treating a cosmetic condition.

Another hormone possibly involved in cellulite formation is progesterone. In some women, it can cause water retention, weight gain, and impaired veins—all of which aggravate cellulite. Further, progesterone, along with estradiol, stimulates fat accumulation in the hips and buttocks.

Progesterone, however, has some merits. Among them, it has the ability to inhibit a family of enzymes that specifically break down collagen. Once more is known regarding this benefit, progesterone may emerge as an important guardian against skin aging.

WATER RETENTION

Medically known as edema, water retention aggravates cellulite by weakening the connective tissue in the skin. Normally, water moves from the capillaries into body tissues, which extract what they need for nourishment. The capillaries then reabsorb the remaining water—a process regulated by the kidneys and controlled by special hormones. Day in and day out, this process continues without incident, maintaining a normal balance of water in our blood and tissues.

But for various reasons, fluid imbalances can occur, resulting in that uncomfortable feeling of puffiness, or water retention. This retention of fluid manifests itself as swelling, which can be generalized, or localized to a specific area of the body. Water dams up in certain places such as the legs, around the eyelids, even in abdominal spaces. You look "fat" even though it's just water weight.

Some of the most common causes of water retention include:

- premenstrual hormonal fluctuations, in which higher ratios of estrogen to progesterone cause the body to stockpile sodium and thus retain excess fluid.
- food sensitivities and allergies, in which swelling and other symptoms occur as an adverse reaction to a specific food. Excess sugar, for example, can promote sodium retention and cause water retention.
- too much salt, which signals the body to dilute the salt by retaining water.
- inadequate water. Paradoxically, water is one of the best preventive measures against fluid retention. Your kidneys need a constant supply of water to properly eliminate fluids and waste products from your body. If water is in short supply, the kidneys tend to hoard water, and bloat can set in.
- protein or thiamin deficiencies in the diet. Thiamin is a B vitamin involved in energy production.
- specific illnesses, including congestive heart failure, kidney disease, underactive thyroid, or varicose veins.
- medications, including prescription appetite suppressants, oral contraceptives, and some antacids.

If a medical problem has been ruled out as the cause of water retention, the condition can be treated naturally—by increasing fluid intake, reducing dietary sugar and sodium, eating diuretic foods such as cranberries and cucumbers, and exercising regularly.

GLYCOSAMINOGLYCANS (GAGS)

Cellulite-affected areas have higher than normal concentrations of glycosaminoglycans (GAGs). Present in connective tissue, GAGs are proteins that bind to water. The increased density of GAGs in cellulite-affected areas causes the skin to soak up water, giving rise to water retention and further weakening the integrity of the connective tissue. This may worsen the appearance of existing cellulite.

POOR MICROCIRCULATION

Impaired circulation may lead to the formation of cellulite. The primary function of the circulatory system is to carry oxygen and nutrients to tissues, and carry away carbon dioxide and other waste products produced by metabolic reactions inside cells.

The system is made up of the heart, blood, and blood vessels. Arteries are the vessels through which oxygen-rich blood is pumped by the heart to every part of the body. Veins are the vessels that carry blood from organs and tissues back to the heart. The heart pumps blood to the lungs to be oxygenated. Arteries and veins are connected by very fine channels called capillaries.

"Microcirculation" refers to the part of the circulatory system made up of capillaries, the smallest blood vessels in the body, and venules, tiny veins connecting capillaries to larger veins. Microcirculation permeates every tissue of the body, transporting nutrients to cells and carrying away waste products.

Microcirculation can become impaired due to inflammation, leaky vessels, sluggish blood flow, and the weakening of blood vessel walls. As a result, oxygen and nutrients do not reach body tissues in quantities substantial enough for normal cellular metabolism. This causes an accumulation of toxic waste products in tissues, which can lead to tissue damage and poor oxygenation. Starved of oxygen and nourishment, the connective tissue in skin develops abnormally. The septa will actually thicken, and as we discovered (see p. 11), this thickening is responsible for the quilted, or mattresslike, appearance that is so characteristic of cellulite.

Another theory has it that cellulite develops when tiny blood vessels in the fat layer become damaged, possibly due to inflammation. Blood circulation slows, and fluid builds up. Both conditions cause the fat layer to swell and the fat within chambers to press out against the septa.

The efficiency at which fat is burned depends on the availability of oxygen. If there is good blood flow to fat tissue, it will be well oxygenated and able to easily liberate stored fat when the body requires it for energy. Impaired microcirculation, however, prevents the liberation of fat from fat cells because there is not enough oxygen around to kindle the process. Fat tissue with poor circulation is hard to budge. A characteristic of cellulite-affected tissue is that it has very poor microcirculation. Increasing microcirculation in those areas through exercise and the use of cellulite control supplements helps rid the body of cellulite and makes the body more cellulite resistant.

FAULTY LYMPHATIC CIRCULATION AND DRAINAGE

Another suspected cause of cellulite is poor lymphatic circulation and drainage in subcutaneous fat. In your body, there is a secondary circulatory system called the lymphatic system. It is an elaborate network of organs, tissues, and vessels whose major functions are to transport digested fat from the intestine to the bloodstream and to defend the body against invasion by disease-causing agents.

Lymph organs include the spleen, which manufactures lymphocytes, a type of white blood cell; the tonsils, which entrap harmful agents that may enter the body through breathing and eating; and Peyer's patches (located in the small intestines), which contain cells that destroy harmful bacteria.

The main lymphatic tissues are lymph nodes, also called lymph glands. Shaped like tiny kidneys, they produce cells called phagocytes, which engulf and destroy infectious and toxic substances. During an infection, the lymph nodes mass-produce phagocytes and become swollen as a result. There are some six hundred lymph nodes in the body.

Lymph vessels include lymphatic capillaries, which connect to larger ducts. Lymph vessels collect and transport a transparent, slightly yellow fluid called lymph. Lymph is filled with disease-fighting white blood cells and is transported in and out of the bloodstream as needed. Lymph being returned to the bloodstream passes through lymph nodes, which filter out and destroy unwanted substances. Lymph also helps return water and protein to the bloodstream.

Every twenty-four hours, some five gallons of lymph move from the bloodstream to tissues in the body. Lymph bathes the cells, provides oxygen and nutrients, and carries waste products and toxins away from the cells.

Unlike arteries, veins, and capillaries, lymph vessels have no pump, and so lymph must be pushed along by the involuntary contractions of the vessels themselves, as well as by the exertion of the body's muscles. Valves prevent lymph from moving backward through the vessels.

Overall, the lymphatic system also works like a drainage system, filtering out cellular wastes, or toxins, and other foreign particles. If the system moves too slowly, some of these wastes can become trapped in fat cells. Quite possibly, this trapped waste inflates fat cells and leads to cellulite. In an intriguing study conducted at Brussels University in Belgium and reported by Dr. Elisabeth Dancey in *The Cellulite Solution* (St. Martin's Press), women with cellulite all suffered from deficiencies of the lymphatic system. Worth mentioning too is that leg skin, where most cellulite is found, has the densest and most extensive lymphatic network in the body.

Various factors can adversely affect lymphatic circulation and drainage. These include inadequate nutrition, lack of exercise, insufficient fluid intake, constipation, exposure to pollutants, and stress. Surgery, trauma, infection, or radiation therapy can also damage the lymph system. Medically termed lymphedema, this damage leads to an accumulation of lymphatic fluid, causing swelling, inflammation, and disability.

Lymphedema in the arms is commonly associated with breast cancer patients and survivors, following a surgical removal or radiation treatment of the lymph nodes. It can occur shortly after an insult to the lymph system, or many years afterward.

Patients who have undergone treatment for cancer in the pelvis or lower extremity, or treatment for Hodgkin's disease, often suffer from lymphedema in the legs.

Reversing and treating the factors that lead to poor lymph circulation often results in less cellulite formation and improvement in the appearance of the skin.

FAT GAIN

It's undeniable: In most cases, cellulite is related to an increase in body fat. Fat gain stems primarily from eating excess calories from fat and sugar, without burning them off. There are two types of fat gain. One is termed "hyperplastic obesity" and involves the development of additional fat cells. Hyperplastic obesity usually begins in childhood and is difficult to treat through diet and exercise. But it can occur later in life too—with excessive weight gain due to overeating and lack of exercise. If you gain fifty pounds or more, for example, fat cells start to multiply, and you've got them forever.

The other type occurs when storage fat cells become stuffed with fat, and enlarge as a result. This condition is technically referred to as hypertrophic obesity, and it usually starts when we are adults. An individual fat cell can swell two to five times its normal size for storage. Enlarged, overstuffed fat cells lead to cellulite. Losing weight, however, causes fat cells to shrink, and minimizes the appearance of cellulite.

FAT DISTRIBUTION

Women naturally carry more fat on their hips and thighs. Not coincidentally, that's where most of our cellulite turns up.

Compounding the problem is that hips and thighs are less willing to give up their fat. To lose 2.2 pounds from your hip region, you'd have to lose nearly thirteen pounds elsewhere, according to scientist Y. G. Illouz, writing in the medical journal *Aesthetic Plastic Surgery*.

Why is lower-body fat so hard to budge?

The reason for this has to do with activities occurring at the cellular level. Fat cell size, for example, is regulated by "receptors" called $alpha_2$ and $beta_1$. Receptors are structures mounted on the surfaces of cells that attach to enzymes and hormones and are stimulated in the process. When the $beta_1$ receptor is stimulated, the activity of a fat-burning enzyme inside the fat cell increases and fat cells shrink. But when the $alpha_2$ receptor is stimulated, fat-burning activity is inhibited. Fat stays inside the cell, further inflating the fat cell. $Alpha_2$ receptors are one of our worst enemies when it comes to burning fat!

Most LFDs (localized fat deposits), the deeper of the two layers of subcutaneous fat, have high $alpha_2$ activity—which further explains why it is so difficult to incinerate this type of fat.

GENETICS

Cellulite runs in families. If your mother has it, you may develop it too. You don't actually inherit cellulite, but rather the tendencies that set the stage for it. For instance, if you have a family history of poor circulation, hormonal imbalances, or obesity, you're at a higher risk of developing cellulite.

Obesity, in particular, is a leading cause of cellulite, and only recently have researchers discovered that the tendency toward obesity is inherited. Of course, where there is obesity, there is usually cellulite.

While there is not a cellulite gene per se, there is a gene called the *ob*. The *ob* gene manufactures a protein hormone called leptin. Leptin is secreted by fat tissue and released into the bloodstream. From there, it travels to the brain. Its job is to help the body regulate its fat stores by curbing appetite and stimulating the metabolism.

Scientists speculate that obese people may be genetically resistant to the effects of leptin. In other words, their brain cells are unresponsive to leptin in much the same way body cells of diabetics are unresponsive to insulin. Research has been under way to develop a leptin-based drug that might overcome this leptin resistance.

Regardless of your genetic fate, there is still much you can do to keep your body cellulite resistant through natural therapies.

AGING

Cellulite becomes more noticeable with age, as the septa, the connective tissue, shrink and the skin holding the fat in place becomes looser and less elastic.

Aging bodies also tend to accumulate more fat. In fact, body fat can double between the ages of twenty and fifty, unless you practice weight control through diet and exercise. Although part of the problem is overeating and underexercising, the body's ability to burn fat decreases with age—a finding that has been verified in a clinical trial.

Investigators at Tufts University in Boston analyzed how sixteen women—half in their twenties, the other half over sixty—burned meals consisting of peanut butter and jelly sandwiches and milk. The portions ranged from a 250-calorie snack to a 1000-calorie meal. Basically, the older women burned only

70 percent as much fat from the larger meal as the younger diners did.

One reason, according to the study, may be that older women have higher levels of glucagon, a hormone that instructs the body to dump more sugar into the blood. A sugar overload restricts the body from burning fat.

The good news is that after ages sixty to seventy, body fat declines in women. Thus, cellulite development may eventually grind to a halt as you enter your golden years.

LIFESTYLE FACTORS

Cellulite has been termed a "lifestyle condition," meaning that our health habits influence it for better or worse. One of the major lifestyle factors affecting the development of cellulite is diet. A high-fat, high-sugar diet, in particular, produces an increase in body fat, and with it, cellulite. Fat from food is chemically similar to fat in the body and thus easy to store. Many studies have shown that overweight people prefer foods higher in fat and sugar.

To elaborate on this point: Let's say you eat 100 extra calories from a fatty food like candy or french fries. Your body may burn just three of those fat calories and stockpile the rest as body fat. In other words, 97 percent of all fat calories are turned into body fat.

But, if you eat 100 additional calories from a natural, complex carbohydrate such as rice or sweet potatoes, you burn 23 of those calories. The rest is put away in the liver or muscles as glycogen (the body's storage form of carbohydrate), awaiting use as energy for activity or exercise. By limiting the amount of fat and eating "good" calories, you can whittle away body fat and minimize cellulite.

Not only does diet affect the development of cellulite, so do diet practices, such as crash dieting or yo-yo dieting. Crash dieting refers to the behavior of eating less than 800 calories a day—a poor dietary habit that can result in an abrupt loss of weight. Sudden weight loss makes it difficult for the skin to normally retract back and conform to the smaller body size. In addition, it stresses the underlying structure of the skin and can intensify cellulite.

Going on and off diets, otherwise known as yo-yo dieting, also promotes the development of cellulite. Women who repeatedly yo-yo diet tend to have higher deposits of fat on their hips and buttocks than those who keep their weight fairly stable.

A second important lifestyle consideration is exercise. Regular physical activity is one of the most important steps you can take to make your body cellulite resistant. Exercise maintains good muscular tone and healthy connective tissue—both of which keep the skin firm and taut. Exercise is also the best defense against unsightly weight gain. Women who are sedentary tend to be heavier, with more cellulite, than women who are regular exercisers.

Smoking aggravates cellulite too. Cigarettes and other tobacco products contain a powerful, addictive drug called nicotine. Nicotine damages microcirculation by causing tiny blood vessels to constrict. Consequently, less blood is able to flow through them. The reduced blood flow damages the walls of the blood vessels. To make matters worse, smoking generates unstable oxygen molecules called free radicals, which do further injury not only to blood vessels, but also to lymph vessels. Free radicals can do irreparable harm to all bodily tissues.

In some women, repeated pregnancies can contribute to the development of cellulite because of the increase in estrogen during pregnancy. Women who are pregnant should maintain excellent nutritional health and not gain more weight than is recommended by their obstetricians. Poor eating habits ultimately affect the health of their children, since the number of fat cells in children is determined by an expectant mother's nutritional state.

Are you a sun worshipper? There's no doubt about it: Having a tan does minimize the appearance of cellulite. But unless you apply a good sunscreen with a sun protection factor (SPF) of 15 or higher, you could be accelerating the development of cellulite. Repeated exposure to sunlight increases the activity of free radicals. In the skin, free radicals damage tissue-producing fibroblasts, decrease normal collagen production, and increase the synthesis of GAGs, which causes the skin to soak up and retain water. In addition, free radical damage promotes the formation of an abnormal type of collagen—one that is quite inelastic. Taken together, these events injure the skin and connective tissue. Skin becomes looser and less elastic, and cellulite, more obvious.

Why There's Hope

The development of cellulite cannot yet be traced to a single cause. Like so many conditions, an interplay of multiple factors is at work. But if you review the causes of cellulite described above, you'll see that, with the exception of aging and genetic factors, most are controllable. That should encourage you. With better personal care, the proper natural treatments, and positive changes in your lifestyle, you can prevent cellulite, minimize its appearance, or stop its progression altogether.

The next chapter gives an overview of the measures you can start taking right now to make your body cellulite resistant. Each of these measures is described in detail in subsequent chapters of this book.

CHAPTER 2

Evaluating Your Cellulite

Cellulite is a progressive condition, meaning it can worsen unless you take steps to halt the process, or at least slow it down. Writing in the medical publication *Journal of Dermatologic Surgery and Oncology*, F. Nürnberger, M.D., and G. Müller, M.D., codified the following four stages of cellulite formation based on thigh and buttocks biopsies of 150 cadavers and thirty living women with cellulite.

Stage 0

Stage 0 describes smooth, cellulite-free skin and is common in many slim women and young girls.

If you're in Stage 0, consider yourself fortunate—at least for now. Should you have a family history of cellulite, however, adopting healthy lifestyle practices early will help prevent the development of cellulite later on.

Stage I

In this stage, the surface of your skin is still relatively smooth while you're standing or lying down. However, your skin may appear slightly dimpled on certain small patches, most notably on the rear of your upper thighs. This is the earliest sign of cellulite development, but its progress can be interrupted at this stage if it is recognized and proper measures are taken.

Stage II

If you let yourself become overweight or obese, cellulite development will probably progress to Stage II. While you're lying down, the surface of your skin appears smooth. But when you stand up, the dimpling is more apparent. Stage II is common in women ages thirty-five to forty.

Stage III

In Stage III, the surface of the skin is dimpled in a lying or standing position. Stage III is very common after menopause and in obesity. Underneath the skin in Stages II and III, there is age-related degradation of collagen and elastin. Both stages are associated with increased deposition of fat.

Size Up Your Figure

The staging descriptions listed above can help you identify whether your cellulite is advanced, or in an early stage. No matter what stage you're in, though, keep in mind that the therapies and preventive techniques now available can rid you of cellulite or at least minimize it—and do it naturally.

In addition to evaluating your cellulite, it's a good idea to size up your overall figure in terms of its "body composition." Essentially, body composition refers to how much body fat and lean muscle you have, and is expressed in percentages.

Having a higher percentage of muscle is desirable because it makes your figure look firm and youthful—and less cellulite-ridden. As I mentioned in the previous chapter, you need a certain amount of essential fat for good health—about 12 to 15 percent. But too much storage fat can affect your appearance, your health, and the development of cellulite. To give you an idea of how much fat is desirable, see Table 2.1 below. It rates body fat percentages from "excellent" to "obese."

There are various methods available to measure weight and body composition. These are discussed below.

- **Scales** are helpful for keeping track of your body weight, which is the combined poundage of your muscles, bones, body water, and fat. But since they register only weight, scales can be misleading. One chief reason is that muscle weighs more than fat. So for a muscular woman, 150 pounds might be perfect. For someone else, this might be dangerously overweight. Plus, if you gain a pound or more, that gain might be lean muscle—exactly what you want for a firm figure.

  A scale provides useful information, but you need an additional measurement of whether you're tubby or toned. A better evaluation of how well you're losing fat is an assessment that tells you the composition of your weight, particularly how much is lean muscle and how much is pure fat. The following techniques are useful for assessing body composition.
- **The skin fold technique** is an excellent way to assess body fat and muscle. It measures fat just under the skin. Skin folds are taken by a set of calipers, a device that

Table 2.1—Body Fat Percentage Ratings

Rating	Women
Excellent	10–15%
Good	16–19%
Acceptable	20–24%
Too fat	25–29%
Obese	30% or more

pinches up folds of fat away from the underlying muscle tissue. The measurements are plugged into a formula that calculates body fat and lean mass percentages. The skin fold technique is a very accurate method for assessing body composition. As many as ten sites may be measured, although the combined measurement of the abdomen, triceps, chest, and thigh skin folds is usually enough for an accurate reading.

- **Ultrasound** is a popular body composition technique. Ultrasound waves pass through the skin and measure underlying fat and muscle. Typically, scans are taken in several areas of the body, then estimated mathematically in a manner similar to skinfold thicknesses. The measurements are used to calculate your body composition. Ultrasound is a simple, painless procedure that takes just five to ten minutes. The results are available immediately after the test.

- **Electrical impedance** involves passing a painless electrical current through the body. The current is introduced at electrodes placed on the hands and feet. Fat tissue won't conduct the current, but fat-free tissue (namely water) will. The faster the current passes through the body, the less body fat there is. Readings obtained from the test are put into special formulas adjusted for height, sex, and age to calculate body fat and fat-free mass percentages.

  Some newer electrical impedance devices resemble bathroom scales, but with electrodes on the pad. You simply step on the pad, and the device measures your body composition instantly. It then displays and prints out your weight, body fat, total body water, and muscle. These devices are very handy and cost about $200 per unit.

- **Circumference measurements,** using a simple tape measure, are a great way to track your body composition. At the same site each time, measure the circumferences of your hips, thighs, and other body parts. Record these numbers and watch them change for the better as you undertake your fat and cellulite reduction program.

The Cellulite Breakthrough Plan

Now that you've assessed your figure, what's next? Instead of simply living with cellulite—and accepting it as cosmetic fate—you can do something about it, once and for all. Although some physicians consider it incurable and not treatable, cellulite can be minimized, and in many cases erased completely, by using a comprehensive five-step approach that combines a variety of techniques. Some of these techniques are common sense, such as diet and exercise. Many others were pioneered in other countries and are just now being introduced in the United States. It's high time we started putting them to use.

Let's take a look at each of the five steps.

Step 1
Consider the use of nutritional supplements, including cellulite control supplements, natural fat burners, and dietary support supplements.

Suppose there were a pill that could magically banish your cellulite. Wouldn't you want to try it?

Good news: There may be such a pill (several in fact)—supplements that contain all-natural ingredients and are obtainable without a doctor's prescription.

The real breakthrough against cellulite involves supplementation with natural formulas containing herbs such as bladderwrack, grape seed extract, sweet clover, and ginkgo that together have a synergistic effect. At least one of these supplements—Cellasene—has impressive clinical research supporting its effectiveness. What's more, Cellasene has been endorsed by leading physicians who specialize in treating cellulite and other skin disorders.

Anticellulite supplements appear to work by strengthening the connective tissue around the fat, improving circulation around the skin and fat, and flushing out retained fluids. If your cellulite is widespread and advanced, you should definitely consider supplementation with a cellulite control product.

In addition, there is a whole other arsenal of natural fat burners that have been clinically proven to help you fight fat, and quite possibly the cellulite that accompanies it. Also, there are other supplements to consider that protect against forces involved in cellulite formation. You can learn about all of these supplements in part II of this book.

Step 2
Follow a healthy, cellulite-fighting diet.

If you lose body fat through diet, cellulite becomes less noticeable. A low-sugar, low-fat, high-fiber, high-protein diet fights cellulite by shrinking fat cells and preventing them from getting fatter. This is the type of diet described in my 30-Day Anticellulite Diet in chapter 8.

Step 3
Exercise regularly, using a combination of strength training, a special type of stretching known as fascial stretching, and aerobics.

Certain types of exercise, including strength training and stretching, tone up muscles and connective tissue underlying the subcutaneous fat. This "irons out" dimply skin, leading to firm-looking hips, thighs, and buttocks. Plus, at sites on the body where muscles are firm, there's decreased fat. But where muscles are untoned, there's usually a lot of fat. Untoned muscles are less metabolically active than firm muscles are. Consequently, they don't burn calories as well, and fat pounds tend to pile on in all the wrong places.

Engaging in dance or vigorous sports produces the same results. Female dancers and athletes with well-toned bodies rarely have cellulite. Further, aerobic exercise such as walking, jogging, or bicycling improves blood circulation to areas of the body where fat is resistant to liberation.

Another point to ponder, especially if you're young or have young daughters: Medical authorities who study cellulite say the best way to prevent it is to avoid weight gain from childhood on. Thus, the key is not letting the spiral of weight gain continue. The best cellulite-fighting moves you can make now are to follow a prudent diet and engage in regular exercise.

Step 4
Optimize your results from supplementation, diet, and exercise by using supportive treatments such as massage and anticellulite creams.

Your thighs can certainly be made smoother, even slimmer, through the use of supportive treatments such as massage and anticellulite creams. Their effects are temporary, however, and these treatments can be costly.

But if you have widespread cellulite and are self-conscious about it, you can derive a lot of satisfaction and cosmetic relief from using supportive treatments.

One of these is Endermologie, a technique that employs a patented machine that was developed in France in the 1970s. A technician moves the machine over your hips, legs, and buttocks, which are covered with a nylon stocking to reduce friction. Endermologie and similar forms of massage help improve circulation, reduce fluid buildup in the tissues, and enhance the removal of waste products. This technique does not rid the body of cellulite but reduces its appearance.

Another type of anticellulite massage is lymphatic massage, performed in the direction of blood flow to help promote lymph circulation and drainage. The goal is to flush out toxins, reduce cellulite, and reduce thigh diameter. This technique does not remove cellulite but instead minimizes the dimply appearance of the skin as fluid buildup in the tissues is reduced.

There are numerous topical agents on the market that temporarily reduce the appearance of cellulite. Designed to be rubbed into the skin, these products claim to produce results through various mechanisms. Some are truly effective, but the benefits cease when the treatment is stopped. Topical agents employed to treat cellulite include methylxanthines, retinoids, lactic acid, herbals, and skin-firming lotions.

Massage and creams are icing on the cake—nice to do for yourself, but not priority treatments for developing a cellulite-resistant body. If all you tried were massage and creams, you'd be disappointed. Your best results will come from a combination of supplementation, diet, and exercise.

Step 5
Maintain a cellulite-resistant body by making permanent changes in your lifestyle.

With so much of today's health advice, it's easy to take it for a while, then discard it and move on to something else. Maintaining a cellulite-resistant body is possible only if you make a lifelong commitment to healthy principles and incorporate them into your daily life.

There are reasons for committing to a healthy lifestyle other than ridding your body of cellulite: You may just get healthier! Just think: You'll be changing your diet, exercising, and taking health-building supplements. All of these changes add up to more than just a cellulite-resistant figure. They add up to a healthier, more vibrant and youthful body.

Aside from less cellulite, here's what else you can potentially expect from following the Cellulite Breakthrough Plan:

- *A leaner, fitter, more cellulite-resistant figure.* You'll start to see visible results as rapidly as the first week of the program.
- *A sky-high metabolism.* Your body becomes a fat-burning machine because you'll be exercising and eating properly to fuel it.
- *Through-the-roof energy levels.* You'll rediscover just how much energy your body can really produce. Physical energy crises will become a thing of the past.
- *Reduced risk for heart disease.* You may think heart disease is a "guy thing"—you know, like football, hunting, or John Wayne movies. But that perception is not only false, it's dangerous. Among women, heart disease claims more

PART I

A Cellulite Primer

lives than all forms of cancer combined, even breast cancer. But once you adopt a healthier lifestyle—one that involves proper nutrition and regular exercise—you reduce your risk because your heart and blood vessels become more efficient at doing their jobs.

- *Reduced risk for breast cancer.* Exercise reduces your chances of getting breast cancer. According to some significant scientific research, women who exercise an average of four hours a week reduce their risk of breast cancer by approximately 50 percent. Those who exercise just one to three hours a week cut their risk by 30 percent.

   The reason for this risk reduction? Scientists speculate that exercise protects breasts by altering hormone levels and decreasing ovulation—two factors known to help guard against breast cancer. The important message here is that lifelong exercise is one possible means of preventing this dreaded disease.

- *Protection against osteoporosis.* No doubt you've heard of osteoporosis. This bone-thinning disease is a debilitating, sometimes fatal disorder, in which vital minerals like calcium leach from your bones as you age. The good news is that strength-training exercises like the ones you'll be doing in this program strengthen the skeleton by stimulating the bone to produce new cells. In addition, a healthy diet plays a pivotal role in preventing or at least slowing down this crippling illness.

- *Stronger immunity and better resistance to disease.* Exercise stimulates the immune system by producing antibodies and virus-fighting cells. Proper nutrition that includes a healthy diet and supplements boosts immunity too.

- *Postponement of the effects of aging.* I'll let you in on a little secret: Aging is accelerated by bad eating habits and inactivity over a lifetime. According to one survey, leading a sedentary life now means about ten years of partial dependency later and a final year of total dependency as your life nears its end. That's certainly nothing to look forward to.

Some incredibly positive news: You can delay, even avoid, many of the pitfalls of aging by taking care of yourself starting right now. The foods you eat, the supplements you take, and the exercises you do are important factors in attaining good health—and maintaining it for a lifetime.

As long as you stick to the cellulite treatment principles outlined in this book, you'll be pleased with the results. A cellulite-resistant body can be yours!

PART II

Anticellulite Supplements

CHAPTER 3

Cellasene: A Supplement Breakthrough

The biggest breakthrough in treating cellulite has been the development of cellulite control supplements. The most well known—and best researched—of these supplements is a product named Cellasene. It has been widely advertised and promoted in the media. In this chapter, I will discuss Cellasene in detail, provide information on its formulation, and explain how to use it.

First, a little background. Cellasene was developed by the Italian pharmaceutical-chemist Gianfranco Merizzi, who was inspired to create the product while judging a Miss Italy pageant. Several contestants, all young and beautiful—but plagued with cellulite—begged him to formulate an anticellulite product, and after intense experimentation Cellasene was born.

The Italian manufacturer of Cellasene is Medestea Internazionale. The product's American distributor is Rexall Sundown, a leading developer, manufacturer, and marketer of vitamins, nutritional supplements, and consumer health products. In a news release prepared on behalf of the two companies, Dr. Merizzi said, "Women around the world are finding

Cellasene can help to eliminate the unsightly problem of cellulite, which cannot be metabolized even when dieting."

Cellasene contains a blend of herbs known to work inside the body to help reduce—and often eliminate—cellulite by modifying the structure and function of the skin. This blend of herbs works to strengthen connective tissue, minimize fluid buildup in tissues, enhance blood flow, and maintain the elasticity of the skin. In other words, Cellasene works to eliminate cellulite at the source of the problem—below the surface of the skin.

Like many herbal supplements, it contains extracts. An extract is a solution prepared by soaking the herb in a solvent. Let's take a closer look at the Cellasene's chief ingredients and what is known about their individual benefits.

Grape Seed Extract

Who would imagine that those tiny, rather annoying seeds we encounter while biting into a juicy grape would yield one of nature's healthiest compounds?

Derived from the common grapevine, grape seeds, when processed, yield an extract loaded with natural health-building agents called procyanidins (also known as oligomeric procyanidins or OPCs).

These remarkable compounds positively influence the appearance of cellulite in several ways. Procyanidins:

- **Help strengthen connective tissue.** Maintaining the structural integrity of connective tissue is key to reducing cellulite. Procyanidins accomplish this in an important way. They preserve connective tissue by interfering with the activity of destructive enzymes that break down the main structural components of connective tissue, namely collagen, elastin, and hyaluronic acid (a natural lubricant in joints and tissues). The net effect is to strengthen and rejuvenate connective tissue below, as well as the skin, for a smoother, firmer appearance above.

- *Improve microcirculation.* Often used in the treatment of microcirculatory disorders, procyanidins may improve blood and oxygen flow by dilating blood vessels. They may also protect capillary walls and promote normal permeability of capillaries. Both actions have a normalizing effect on surrounding tissues.

  Improving microcirculation is important in reducing cellulite. Some medical authorities have theorized that faulty or slow circulation may promote the formation of fat. Where there is decreased circulation in the body, there is often a corresponding increase in fatty tissue. By the same token, in areas of ample blood flow, there is less fat.

- *Reduce fluid accumulation.* Procyanidins have the power to reduce fluid buildup in tissues and have thus been used to treat lymphedema, a chronic disorder characterized by persistent swelling in the arms or legs due to blocked lymph channels.

- *Fight free radicals.* Procyanidins may also act as potent antioxidants. Antioxidants are nutrients that protect cell membranes from the onslaught of free radicals, the unstable oxygen molecules mentioned earlier. Free radicals wreak molecular havoc by boring through cell walls and making it easy for bacteria, viruses, and other disease-causing agents to slip in and do often-irreparable harm. Some experts feel that free radical damage to blood vessel walls promotes the development of cellulite. Procyanidins may help protect blood vessels from this type of injury. These nutrients have also been found to bolster the power of another antioxidant, vitamin C, and extend its lifetime.

  There seems to be no end to the amazing power of procyanidins. The grape seed extract used in Cellasene has been complexed, or specially bonded, with phospholipids for better absorption and use by the body. Phospholipids are fat-related substances that can react with both water and fats.

  The grape seed extract in Cellasene is part of the

product's proprietary blend, along with bladderwrack extract, sweet clover extract, and *Ginkgo biloba* extract. Three soft gels of Cellasene contain 702 milligrams of this proprietary blend.

Bladderwrack

Used in steam baths by Native Americans to treat joint problems and other illnesses, bladderwrack is a brown alga rich in iodine, a mineral required by the body in tiny amounts and an essential component of thyroid hormones.

Because it contains iodine, bladderwrack is thought to correct a sluggish thyroid, thus boosting the metabolism to treat obesity. Bladderwrack is a familiar homeopathic weight loss formula in Europe and has been available in American health food stores for several years now.

Bladderwrack also contains a carbohydrate called fucoidan, which exerts a mild anticlotting action and acts as an anti-inflammatory agent. Scientific studies suggest that the fucoidan in bladderwrack enhances circulation and helps alleviate localized inflammation.

Ginkgo Biloba Extract

Ginkgo, derived from the leaves of an ornamental tree, improves and normalizes blood circulation to the skin, extremities, and brain. It accomplishes this by thinning the blood, enhancing the health and tone of blood vessels, inhibiting abnormal clotting, and fighting fluid buildup. These actions have been extensively verified by numerous clinical trials.

Ginkgo also protects against oxidative damage that normally occurs as our bodies burn oxygen to live. If not held in check by antioxidants, oxidation can corrode cell membranes in much the same way rust forms on metal. A product of oxidation is free radicals, those nasty molecules that attack bodily tissues.

The multiple talents of ginkgo provide important benefits in reducing cellulite. Because of its antiinflammatory actions, ginkgo could yield additional benefits in reducing the tissue swelling often associated with cellulite.

In the German Commission E monographs, ginkgo is listed as an approved herb for improving microcirculation. The German Commission E is Germany's equivalent to our Food and Drug Administration (FDA), and its monographs are a clinical reference tool describing scores of herbs and their therapeutic applications.

Sweet Clover Extract

We naturally equate clover, or shamrock, with good luck. But if you want to get lucky in minimizing cellulite, check out sweet clover instead of shamrock.

Sweet clover contains a beneficial constituent called coumarin, known to reduce lymphedema of the arms and legs. Coumarin has been used to flavor foods and candies, and because of its sweet smell, it has been employed as a fragrance in cosmetics.

The German Commission E has approved sweet clover for treating lymphatic congestion and problems arising from chronic venous insufficiency, a condition associated with both varicose veins and phlebitis, the inflammation of a vein.

The daily dose of coumarin from sweet clover in the initial three softgel per day recommended dosage of Cellasene is ten to 11 milligrams daily—well within the safe, effective three- to 30-milligram dosage window recommended by the German Commission E.

Fish Oil

For more than twenty-five years, research reports have been pouring in about the potent health benefits of fish oils, namely omega-3 fatty acids, found primarily in deep-sea fish. There are nonfish sources too, and these include flaxseed oil, canola oil, and soybean oil. The two most beneficial members of the omega-3 family are eicosapentaenoic acid (EPA) and docosa-hexanoic acid (DHA).

Their healthful properties first came to light when scientists discovered that Eskimos have a lower rate of heart disease and stroke than other populations do, despite their high-fat diet. The difference is that Eskimos eat twenty times more fish than Americans do, and fish is full of omega-3 fatty acids.

Because of this link, omega-3 fatty acids have become best known for their ability to promote cardiovascular health. They have been found to lower blood pressure, reduce cholesterol, thwart dangerous blood clotting, and protect against irregular heartbeats.

Your body uses omega-3 fatty acids to produce prostaglandins. Prostaglandins are hormonelike biochemicals that trigger many processes in the body. Among other duties, prostaglandins help reduce inflammation.

There are not-so-friendly prostaglandins in the body too, which are involved in producing inflammation. But in a rather dramatic nutritional rescue, omega-3 fatty acids interfere with their manufacture by grabbing on to an enzyme that harmful prostaglandins need for production. The net effect is a reduction in inflammation.

The medical literature suggests that inflammation plays a role in the development of cellulite, or that changes in the connective tissue cause inflammation, which leads to cellulite. Accordingly, supplementation with fish oil could help reduce cellulite-associated inflammation.

The fish oil in Cellasene is part of the product's Support Blend, along with borage seed oil and soya lecithin (see below). Three softgels of Cellasene contain 1230 milligrams of the Support Blend.

Borage Seed Oil

The borage plant has been a popular herb since ancient times, when the Romans claimed it bestowed courage and banished depression. Today, the herb is best known for its oil, pressed from the seeds of the plant.

Borage seed oil is high in gamma-linolenic acid (GLA), an omega-6 fatty acid. Like the omega-3 fatty acids, GLA exerts an antiinflammatory effect in the body.

Soya Lecithin

Cellasene also contains the phospholipid lecithin. Lecithin is found in nervous tissue, primarily the myelin sheath (the protective covering for the nerves); in egg yolk, soybeans, and corn; and as an essential constituent of animal and vegetable cells. Lecithin is the richest source of choline, a nutrient that prevents fats from building up in the liver and aids the body in metabolizing cholesterol.

The lecithin used in Cellasene is derived from soy, one of nature's healthiest food sources.

The Science Behind Cellasene

Unlike some dietary supplements, Cellasene has been tested scientifically to prove that it does indeed minimize the appearance of cellulite. To date, there have been two clinical trials and one pilot study conducted on Cellasene.

THE CLINICAL STUDIES

The first two trials were conducted in Italy at the University of Pavia NonInvasive Diagnostic Clinic, Policlinico San Matteo Hospital. All the participants were healthy adult women of various ages and weights. During the studies, they did not use any other anticellulite oral or topical preparations. Their diets and exercise levels remained constant throughout the studies.

Prior to each investigation, the researchers measured the circumference of the women's hips, right thigh, and right ankle using a tape measure. Their subcutaneous fatty tissue layer was measured by ultrasound and skinfold testing. Both methods are accurate, well-accepted techniques for assessing body fat.

The first study involved twenty-five women, with an average age of thirty-eight. They supplemented with Cellasene for eight weeks and followed the normal prescribed doses.

By the end of the experimental period, in September 1997, positive changes had occurred in the women's body circumferences. These are listed in Table 3.1.

As you can tell, the circumference of the women's hips and thighs was pared down rather significantly—by more than half an inch. The thickness of their fatty tissue layer was reduced too; this reduction was measured by both calipers and by ultrasound. Measured by a Doppler device, microcirculation in the skin increased as well.

The second study involved forty women, divided into a placebo group of fifteen and a Cellasene group of twenty-five.

Table 3.1—Study 1

Measurement	Average Initial Measure	Average Final Measure	Average Differences
Hip circumference	98.2 cm (38.66 in)	96.9 cm (38.14 in)	1.3 cm (.52 in)
Thigh circumference	57.9 cm (22.8 in)	56.4 cm (22.2 in)	1.5 cm (.6 in)
Ankle circumference	21.9 cm (8.62 in)	21.4 cm (8.43 in)	.5 cm (.19 in)
Reduction in fatty tissue layer as measured by calipers (mm)	*6.0 mm (0.24 in)*	*5.5 mm (0.22 in)*	*.5 mm (0.02 in)*
Reduction in fatty tissue layer as measured by ultrasound (thickness units)	6.9	6.4	.5

Adapted from: Medestea Internazionale, S.R.L., and Rexall Sundown, Inc. 1999. Expert scientific paper on Cellasene. May, 33.

Table 3.2—Study 2

Measurement	Average Initial Measure	Average Final Measure	Average Difference
Hip circumference	97.1 cm (38.22 in)	94.8 cm (37.32 in)	2.3 cm (.9 in)
Thigh circumference	56.6 cm (22.28 in)	54.9 cm (21.61 in)	1.7 cm (.67 in)
Reduction in fatty tissue layer as measured by calipers (mm)	5.3 mm (0.21 in)	4.7 mm (0.19 in)	.6 mm (0.02 in)
Reduction in fatty tissue layer as measured by ultrasound (thickness units)	5.9	5.6	.3

Adapted from: Medestea Internazionale, S.R.L., and Rexall Sundown, Inc. 1999. Expert scientific paper on Cellasene. May, 36.

The average age of the volunteers was 33.9 years. In addition to measuring circumference and fatty layer dimensions, the researchers took blood pressure and blood lipid measurements before and after the study.

As shown in Table 3.2, the results of the second study highlight Cellasene's powerful effects: The Cellasene supplementers lost significant girth from their hips and thighs. Microcirculation in the thigh surface increased as well. The placebo group, however, had no comparable results.

In addition, blood pressure was slightly reduced in the Cellasene group, but not in the placebo group. There were no significant changes in the blood fat profiles of either group.

After reviewing this research, independent experts agreed that the most critical parameter in evaluating the effectiveness of the supplement was the thigh measurement. Here's why: Ankles are more likely to retain water, so it's hard to get an accurate reading of fat tissue reduction, while hips are subject to variables in measurements that are affected by the position and posture of the subject.

Further, the Italian studies demonstrated that Cellasene reduced cellulite in women's thighs and hips in approximately 90 percent of the subjects.

Both of these studies have been reviewed by outside independent experts credentialed in nutrition, dermatology, and cellulite. These experts include scientific and medical doctors who have worked for the U.S. federal government as expert scientific consultants. They concluded that the clinical studies on Cellasene were well designed and adequately controlled.

One of the experts, Peter Pugliese, M.D., a leading authority on cellulite, wrote in a scientific paper on Cellasene: "Based on that review, I conclude that there is adequate evidence that proves that Cellasene eliminates or helps eliminate cellulite, reduces, and works at the source of the problem. I have also determined that Cellasene is a safe dietary supplement, under the ordinary conditions of use set forth in its labeling."

The research may thus be counted on to support the safety and effectiveness of Cellasene to help eliminate cellulite.

THE PILOT STUDY

So positive and encouraging were the Italian studies that additional research has been undertaken. A recent pilot study was performed in New York City by George Beraka, M.D. The duration of the investigation was twelve weeks and involved ten women, with an average age of 35.3 years and an average weight of 127 pounds. They took one Cellasene softgel three times a day for eight weeks. In the final four weeks, they supplemented with one softgel each day.

All women in the trial had cellulite present. After eight weeks of Cellasene supplementation, study participants had an average decrease in thigh circumference of approximately 2.2 cm (just under 1 inch) on each thigh. They maintained this reduction during the four-week maintenance period that followed the initial eight weeks of treatment.

Similar results were observed in skin fold thickness, with a substantial reduction occurring during the initial eight-week treatment phase. Nine subjects (90 percent) reduced their skin fold thickness by approximately 1.5 inches. Hip circumference decreased as well, by just more than half an inch.

The appearance of cellulite was improved as well. Prior to the study, Dr. Beraka had assessed cellulite on each subject, while standing, according to the following scale:

> 0 = no visible cellulite
> 1 = minimal cellulite
> 2 = moderate cellulite
> 3 = marked cellulite
> 4 = severe cellulite

After twelve weeks, three participants experienced a reduction of two grades of cellulite, and five subjects had a reduction of one grade, for a total of 80 percent of the ten participants improving at least one grade. Of the women with an improved cellulite grade, two attained a grade 0, or no visible cellulite, by week twelve. Two women maintained the same grade of cellulite. No subject experienced a worsening of her cellulite grade during the study.

Again, these are encouraging results and indicate that supplementation is an important natural therapy in treating cellulite. In a news release, Dr. Beraka praised Cellasene: "The potential for Cellasene is so great that I am committed to using Cellasene in my Manhattan practice with patients. It's the first product I've ever heard of that is ingested and which apparently attacks cellulite systematically from the inside out."

One of the women who participated in Dr. Beraka's trial was quoted in a May 1999 news release as saying, "I eat healthy and I'm a very active person, but I still had a problem with cellulite on the back of my legs. I'm convinced Cellasene has helped improve the texture of my skin and I've already lost over a half inch in circumference in my upper thigh and still have four weeks to go in the study."

How to Take Cellasene

Without a doubt, Cellasene is an exciting supplement. The question is: How much should you take?

In the initial eight weeks, supplement with three softgels a day with food, according to directions on the label. All three softgels can be taken with meals, if you prefer. For the next nine to sixteen weeks, follow the maintenance program of one softgel daily taken with food. The manufacturer notes that the start-up and maintenance periods may be repeated as needed.

You should not exceed the recommended dosage.

How Long to See Results?

According to the manufacturer, you should notice smoother-feeling legs and firmer tone after eight weeks of continuous use as directed.

It is important to emphasize that Cellasene works in about 90 percent of the women who use it as recommended. In the rest, it may not work, even when taken as directed.

Cellasene and Diet

While supplementing with Cellasene, you needn't go on an overly stringent diet. However, if you eat anything you want without regard to calories or fat intake or without exercising, you will only gain weight, and your cellulite could worsen.

Your best bet is to follow a moderate well-balanced but low-fat diet plan. See chapter 7 for nutritional suggestions that can maximize your results from supplementation.

In addition, drink eight to ten full glasses of water daily to help flush toxins from your body.

A Safe History of Cellasene Use Worldwide

Cellasene has a history of safe and effective use worldwide, according to the manufacturer and distributor. More than 6.5 million units have been sold over a period of six years, with no adverse reports relating to thyroid problems, blood thinning, or other illnesses. Further, the ingredients in Cellasene are commonly used dietary ingredients and enjoy a safe history of use in the United States and around the world.

A cautionary point: Cellasene is formulated with bladderwrack extract, which is high in iodine. The recommended dietary allowance (RDA) for iodine is 150 micrograms daily—which you easily consume by salting your food with less than half a teaspoon of iodized salt. The typical Western diet includes approximately 300 to 400 micrograms of iodine daily, and intakes of 1000 micrograms are considered safe for most adults. Three softgels of Cellasene contain 720 micrograms of iodine—still within safe levels.

It is only at levels of more than 2000 micrograms, however, that iodine becomes quite toxic. Overconsumption of iodine can cause an enlarged thyroid gland and disrupt the normal functioning of thyroid hormones.

Cellasene also contains ginkgo and sweet clover. Theoretically, both have possible blood-thinning properties and should not be taken in conjunction with prescription blood thinners. Nor should you take Cellasene if you have a known allergic reaction to any of its ingredients.

Accordingly, the product carries the following warnings: "Bladderwrack extract contains iodine, and total iodine intake may exceed recommended levels when taking this product. If you suffer from a thyroid condition or if you are taking blood-thinning medication or other medications, consult your health care professional before using this product. Cellasene should not be taken when pregnant or nursing."

Unlike prescription medicines, nutritional supplements such as Cellasene aren't approved by the FDA. Under the Dietary Supplement Health and Education Act of 1994, supplement manufacturers can make nutrition support statements about their products—statements that describe how a product functions in the body. Cellasene's package, for example, says, "Helps Eliminate Cellulite."

But they aren't allowed to claim that the product can treat or cure any disease. Also, supplement labels must carry the following disclaimer: "This statement has not been evaluated by the Food and Drug Administration. This product is not intended to diagnose, treat, cure, or prevent any disease."

Keep in mind that natural supplements such as Cellasene are derived from food or herbs—and thus work *with* your body, rather than against it (as many prescription medicines do). It's always preferable to try the gentlest agent first.

Cellasene and Quality Control

Many people considering supplementation are concerned not only about the safety of a particular supplement, but also about its quality. Is the supplement quality-tested? Does it contain what's on the label? Does it meet acceptable standards?

At present, there are few controls on what goes into supplements, or whether products are even as pure as they should be. That's because herbs are considered food additives, not drugs, and therefore they are not scrutinized by the FDA as drugs are.

Good news about Cellasene: It is subject to strict quality assurance and quality control testing. It is manufactured in Italy at an established pharmaceutical facility and subject to rigorous analytical tests by its U.S. distributor, Rexall Sundown. Prior to release of any Cellasene, Rexall Sundown performs its own independent quality control analyses using both an independent facility and its own in-house laboratory.

Lots of Cellasene are tested and analyzed to confirm that:

- it is free of microbiological contamination.
- iodine levels meet specifications and do not exceed label claims.
- it meets United States Pharmacopeia (USP) standards. The USP is an organization that sets quality standards for supplements, over-the-counter drugs, and prescription medicines.
- it meets all physical specifications for color and weight.

Where Can I Find Cellasene?

Cellasene can be purchased from a variety of sources, including food stores, drugstores, mass market retailers such as Wal-Mart or Kmart, and health food stores.

The product comes in a distinctive pink box. The cost may vary from store to store, but the purchase price is generally $30 for thirty softgels.

You don't need a prescription for Cellasene, but as always, speak to your physician before taking supplements.

CHAPTER 4

Other Cellulite Control Supplements

The introduction of Cellasene in 1998 in the United States created such an international phenomenon that many other anticellulite dietary supplements were launched shortly thereafter. As a consumer interested in eliminating cellulite, you should be familiar with some of these products, particularly with their ingredients, so as to make informed choices when buying supplements.

It is extremely important to read the labels of any anticellulite supplements and to educate yourself about the ingredients they contain and what they can and cannot do. What follows is a description of some anticellulite supplements, their ingredients, and how to use them. This information can serve as a handy reference to consult before making any purchases.

Celite Complex 75

Celite Complex 75 was researched and developed by Jamieson Laboratories of Canada. It is a synergistic formula of biologically active plant extracts from fruits and herbs. These extracts contain nutritional agents that may help fight cellulite and promote healthy microcirculation. In addition, the extracts are formulated in amounts considered safe by herbalists. Each dose of Celite Complex 75 contains ginkgo (250 milligrams), which was discussed in the previous chapter. Other active ingredients in the formulation include the following.

CITRUS BIOFLAVONOIDS

Bioflavonoids, also known as vitamin P, are naturally occurring pigments found in fruits and vegetables. Procyanidins, such as those found in grape seed extract, belong to the bioflavonoid family.

Sources of bioflavonoids include lemons, grapefruit, grapes, plums, apricots, buckwheat, cherries, and blackberries. The bioflavonoids in Celite Complex 75 are derived from citrus fruits.

Bioflavonoids are essential for the proper absorption of vitamin C. When taken together, bioflavonoids and vitamin C are more effective than vitamin C used alone. Bioflavonoids team up with vitamin C to maintain the health of collagen. They also help strengthen the capillaries and regulate their permeability. There are 100 milligrams of citrus bioflavonoids in each dose of Celite Complex 75.

BILBERRY EXTRACT

Bilberry is the European version of the American blueberry. Although commonly used in pies and jellies, bilberry has become an important medicinal herb worldwide. Extracts of the berry can perform some amazing feats—all with relevance to cellulite. The extract contains disease-fighting antioxidants that help protect cells in the walls of the capillaries and increase their flexibility. This allows more oxygen-carrying red blood cells to reach the tissues. Also, the extract stimulates new capillary formation. In short, bilberry extract is an important herb for enhancing microcirculation.

Bilberry extract significantly improves the symptoms of

varicose veins too, including calf and ankle swelling. It also has proven to be beneficial in treating hardening of the arteries, or atherosclerosis. The extract appears to prevent plaque from building up in the arteries.

Bilberry is a German Commission E–approved herb. There are 750 milligrams of bilberry in each dose of Celite Complex 75.

CINNAMON

Cinnamon is everyone's favorite spice, derived from a tree of the laurel family. In addition to flavoring foods, cinnamon is used as a medicine—to treat nausea, relieve stomach gas, and calm fevers. In one scientific experiment, the spice was found to help the body better digest sweets by improving the ability of insulin to move sugar into cells. It has been described as an herbal lipotropic. Technically, "lipotropic" refers to any substance that decreases the rate at which fat is stored in liver cells and accelerates the rate at which fat is dismantled into water, carbon dioxide, and energy during metabolism.

A few natural weight loss supplements contain traces of cinnamon, which is a German Commission E–approved herb. The cinnamon used in Celite Complex 75 is oil of Madagascar cinnamon (20 milligrams).

SEA KELP EXTRACT

Similar to bladderwrack, kelp is a nutritious sea vegetable rich in iodine. Iodine is a trace mineral that helps the thyroid gland produce thyroxin, the principal thyroid hormone involved in metabolism. Each dose of Celite Complex 75 contains 25 milligrams of sea kelp extract.

BROMELAIN

Found naturally in pineapple, bromelain is a proteolytic enzyme, meaning that it is capable of breaking down protein. It is also believed to have strong fat-dissolving properties. For these reasons, it is often recommended as a digestive aid and is found as an ingredient in meat tenderizers.

Bromelain inhibits the action of inflammation-producing substances and is therefore beneficial as an antiinflammatory agent. In addition, bromelain is helpful in reducing edema. It also exhibits some anticlotting properties. The German Commission E has approved bromelain for the treatment of certain types of swelling.

Each dose of Celite Complex 75 is formulated with 100 milligrams of bromelain enzyme.

KOLA NUT EXTRACT

Kola nut extract comes from the seed of an African tree. One of its key constituents is caffeine, which helps your body metabolize fat for fuel. Kola nut is considered a stimulant herb because of its caffeine content and is thus used in numerous supplements marketed as natural pick-me-ups. In fact, the German Commission E has approved kola nut for treating physical and mental fatigue. Kola nut is also an ingredient in many herb-based anticellulite creams.

There are 250 milligrams of kola nut extract in each dose of Celite Complex 75.

SUPPLEMENTING WITH CELITE COMPLEX 75

Jamieson Laboratories, the manufacturer of Celite Complex 75, advises taking two capsules daily with morning or midday meals. Celite is not recommended for expecting or lactating mothers.

There are sixty gelcaps in each bottle, and the product costs approximately $30. You can order it by calling 1–800–247–4499. The manufacturer does not state how long it takes to see results.

CellaFree

CellaFree is manufactured by Bodyonics and sold at health food stores and other outlets through the United States. The supplement is formulated with bladderwrack, grape seed extract, sweet clover extract, ginkgo, fish oils, borage oil, and soya lecithin—all discussed in the previous chapter. Six capsules contain 1000 milligrams of various herbs and fatty acids in amounts considered safe by herbalists.

Consumer information on the label notes: "The exact mechanisms underlying the interference of CellaFree's active ingredients with fat synthesis and deposition remain unclear. However, numerous studies demonstrate that these ingredients regulate various steps in fat accumulation both before and after absorption."

In addition to the ingredients listed above, CellaFree contains the following.

EVENING PRIMROSE OIL

Evening primrose oil comes from a plant that grows wild along roadsides. It is so named because its yellow flowers resemble in color real primroses, and these flowers open only in the evening.

Extracted from the seeds of the plant, evening primrose oil is an excellent natural source of gamma-linolenic acid (GLA), a building block of prostaglandins that help reduce inflammation.

GLA is also involved in weight loss. In fact, people with GLA deficiencies tend to produce more fat in their bodies. Supplementing with evening primrose oil has helped them lose weight.

Research has found that evening primrose oil works best if you are more than 10 percent above your ideal weight. In some people, it promotes weight loss without reducing caloric intake. It is also believed to help rev up the metabolism, so that you burn more calories. Evening primrose oil also helps reduce fluid retention.

OLIGOPEPTIDES

Oligopeptides are natural peptides (partially digested proteins) made from wheat protein. These special forms of wheat protein have been found to help regulate fat deposition and support weight loss in humans, according to information issued by the makers of CellaFree.

CHITOSAN

Chitosan, also known as chitin, is an animal fiber derived from the outer shells of crab and shrimp cells. It is a waste product of the crabbing and shrimping industry that is also used to make glucosamine, a popular natural remedy for arthritis.

As a natural weight loss supplement, chitin is marketed as a "fat binder," meaning that it prevents fat absorption in the stomach by attracting fat and entrapping its molecules. This makes the fat molecules too large to be absorbed through the walls of the gastrointestinal tract. As a result, they are excreted from the bowel without being completely digested. By reducing the amount of fat absorbed by the body, chitosan theoretically helps in weight control.

People allergic to shrimp and other shellfish should discuss the pros and cons of chitosan supplementation with their physicians.

The chitosan in CellaFree is combined with vegetable pulp and citrus pectin from grapefruit. Six capsules of CellaFree contain 1750 milligrams of this blend of fibers, including the oligopeptides.

YERBA MATÉ

Yerba maté is a South American plant whose leaves are dried and made into tea or put into capsules. The herb contains vitamins A, B-complex, C, and the minerals calcium, magnesium, and iron.

Yerba maté is well endowed with caffeine, known to help mobilize fat from storage depots. For that reason, the herb is a fairly common ingredient in natural weight loss supplements and may be helpful against cellulite.

Yerba maté also has a mild diuretic effect. As with any diuretic, supplementing with it may produce temporary water weight loss.

UVA URSI

This herb is derived from the leaves of the bearberry, an evergreen plant. A mild diuretic, uva ursi's active ingredients are ursolic acid and isoquercetin, two natural chemicals that increase urine output. Supplementing with uva ursi promotes loss of excess fluids in tissues, reducing bloat and water retention. Minimizing fluid buildup may help improve the appearance of cellulite.

The German Commission E has approved uva ursi for the treatment of inflammatory disorders of the urinary tract. Six capsules of CellaFree contain a 1000-milligram combination of uva ursi and yerba maté.

SUPPLEMENTING WITH CELLAFREE

Each bottle of CellaFree contains 180 tablets and costs approximately $25. According to the instructions on the label, take two tablets with an eight-ounce glass of water three times daily, preferably with meals.

The manufacturer lists the following caution on the label: "Prior to use, obtain advice from your health care practitioner if you are pregnant or nursing. Keep out of reach of children. Do not consume this product if you suffer from high blood pressure, prostatic hypertrophy, hyperthyroidism, glaucoma, cardiac arrhythmias, or pheochromocytoma. This product should not be consumed in combination with MAO (monoamine oxidase) inhibitors or with any antidepressant drug which blocks the transport of norepinephrine. Curtail or discontinue use if nervousness, sleeplessness or nausea occurs. Not intended for persons under the age of 18. Fucus extract contains a small amount of iodine—if you suffer from hyperthyroidism, you should consult your doctor first."

Cellulite Control

Sold at health food stores and other outlets, Cellulite Control is manufactured by Irwin Naturals and was formulated by a naturopathic physician. It combines the herbs horse chestnut seed extract and gotu kola (see below). According to promotional literature from the manufacturer, this combination has been clinically verified to reduce cellulite.

The product also contains *Ginkgo biloba* (90 milligrams), discussed in the previous chapter. Other herbs in the formula include hawthorn berry, horsetail, ginger root, milk thistle, and cayenne pepper. Here is a closer look at how these ingredients work.

GOTU KOLA

A member of the parsley family, gotu kola is a common weed, usually found growing in drainage ditches in Asia, and in orchards in Hawaii.

A known effect of this herb is that it fights water retention by helping the body eliminate excess fluid. It is also a central nervous system stimulant and believed to be a lipotropic, or fat-burning, herb.

Gotu kola has cellulite-fighting powers: It strengthens the connective tissue between veins to help improve the underlying integrity of the skin. What's more, the herb regenerates normal collagen and reduces the formation of an inelastic type of collagen found in sun-damaged skin.

Two capsules of Cellulite Control contain 400 milligrams of gotu kola extract, which is considered a safe dosage by herbalists.

HORSE CHESTNUT

Processed from the seeds of the chestnut fruit, horse chestnut extract is an effective treatment for varicose veins, a condition in which the veins can't move blood efficiently, or the valves in veins fail to close properly. Consequently, blood tends to congregate, usually in the legs. Vein and capillaries swell, leaking blood and fluid into nearby tissue. Veins near the surface of the skin bulge and meander in corkscrewlike trails.

Horse chestnut extract strengthens vein walls, improves leg vein circulation, and prevents swelling. Its active constituent is aescin. Aescin has been shown in lab dishes to block the activity of the enzyme that breaks down elastin, an important structural fiber in body tissues, including veins. Preserving the elastic tissue of veins aids in the return of blood from the legs to the heart and helps reduce leg swelling.

In addition, horse chestnut seed extract may be a very important herb in protecting against the structural degradation of connective tissue believed to be a factor in cellulite. Horse chestnut extract also acts as an antiinflammatory.

Horse chestnut seed is approved by the German Commission E in dosages of 250 to 312.5 milligrams twice a day for the treatment of chronic venous insufficiency, night cramps in the calves, and swelling of the legs. There are 30 milligrams of horse chestnut seed extract in each two-capsule dose of Cellulite Control.

Cellulite Control also contains horse chestnut root bark (180 milligrams in each two-capsule dose), which is another portion of the plant used medicinally.

HAWTHORN BERRY

Hawthorn preparations are made from the flowers, leaves, or berries of a thorny plant grown in Europe. In Germany and other parts of Europe, hawthorn extracts are widely prescribed to treat heart problems, high blood pressure, and arthritis. Preparations from the hawthorn leaf with flower are approved by the German Commission E. The herb is usually sold in capsule form, and included as an ingredient in natural weight loss supplements.

Studies show that the herb dilates coronary arteries, thus improving blood flow and oxygen supply to the heart.

There are 90 milligrams of hawthorn berries in each two-capsule dose of Cellulite Control. This dosage is well within the safe limits recommended by herbalists.

HORSETAIL

A close relative to a tree that grew in dinosaur days, this herb is a rich source of the trace mineral silicon. Silicon is involved in tissue repair and helps strengthen the walls of arteries and veins.

Herbalists recommend horsetail to treat a wide range of conditions, including kidney problems and bladder disorders. Horsetail acts as a diuretic—which is why the herb is used in natural weight loss supplements and cellulite control products.

The German Commission E has approved horsetail for treating edema. Each two-capsule dose of Cellulite Control is formulated with 64 milligrams of horsetail.

CELLULITE CONTROL PROPRIETARY BLEND

Cellulite Control (two capsules) contains a safe, 136-milligram dose of a proprietary blend of various herbs.

Ginger Root

Used since ancient times, this herb is processed from the underground stem of a tropical plant native to Asia. It is available in tablets, capsules, tea, extracts, syrups, and as an ingredient in some natural weight loss supplements.

Ginger root, which contains a number of beneficial chemicals, has a long list of bona fide medical uses: relieving intestinal gas, treating nausea caused by motion sickness, and reducing inflammation, to name just a few. It is a German Commission E–approved herb for treating motion sickness.

Milk Thistle

Derived from a weedlike plant grown in the Mediterranean area, this herb has been used as a liver protectant since ancient times. The liver is an organ that helps metabolize fat.

For more than sixty years, mounds of research have confirmed milk thistle's benefit on liver health. Most supplements contain standardized extracts of the herb's active ingredient, silymarin, and are used to treat cirrhosis, hepatitis, and other liver diseases, particularly in Europe. In fact, milk thistle is a German Commission E–approved herb for treating liver ailments.

Where weight loss is concerned, milk thistle is thought to be an herbal lipotropic that helps remove fatty substances from the liver.

Cayenne

Capsicum is the red pepper with which you spice your foods. It contains a number of active chemicals and is available as a condiment, in powder form, and as a cream applied topically to relieve joint pain. The German Commission E has approved it as an external treatment for muscle spasms.

Capsicum is added to natural weight loss products because it is believed to stimulate the metabolism by creating heat. You've probably noticed this yourself. After you eat hot spicy foods, your body will heat up. When body heat rises, so does metabolism, and more calories are burned. At least one study has measured the metabolic rates of people who ate capsicum with meals. When a teaspoon of red pepper sauce and a teaspoon of mustard were added to meals, metabolic rates rose by as much as 25 percent.

SUPPLEMENTING WITH CELLULITE CONTROL

According to the manufacturer, you should take one or two capsules up to three times daily with one full glass of water. The product costs approximately $16.50 for a three-week supply of sixty capsules.

The manufacturer has posted the following warning on the label: "Do not use if safety seal on bottle is broken. Check with your doctor before beginning any new weight-loss program. Do not use if you take any MAO inhibitors or if you are pregnant or lactating. Keep out of reach of children. Store in a cool dry place."

Cell Pill

Distributed by Neways International, the Cell Pill is designed to diminish the appearance of cellulite and enhance circulatory health.

Each dose is formulated with various cellulite control herbs, including evening primrose oil (520 milligrams), fish oil (534 milligrams), grape seed extract (5446 milligrams), sweet clover extract (3.6 milligrams), ginkgo (700 milligrams), bladderwrack (600 milligrams), horse chestnut (750 milligrams), and gotu kola (150 milligrams). It also contains some lecithin and a concentrate of juniper berry, an herb commonly used to flavor gin. Juniper berry acts as a diuretic. It has been approved by the German Commission E for treating indigestion. There are 80 milligrams of juniper berry in each dose of Cell Pill.

SUPPLEMENTING WITH CELL PILL

The manufacturer's dosage recommendations advise taking four capsules daily—two in the morning and two in the evening, with food. For a more "intense" program, you can take four in the morning and four in the evening, with food. Although herbal dosages in this supplement are considered safe by herbalists, the manufacturer cautions that people with a thyroid condition or taking blood-thinning or heart medications should consult their physicians before supplementing.

Cell Pill costs approximately $84 for 120 capsules. You can order it through any independent Neways distributor.

Cellu-Rid

Formulated by Biotech Corporation, the ingredients in Cellu-Rid are designed to promote vasodilation (the widening of blood vessels), accelerate fat-burning, and enhance excretion of waste products and excess fluid.

Each capsule of the formulation includes kelp (33 milligrams), uva ursi (five milligrams), juniper berries (five milligrams), soya lecithin (16 milligrams) and a special blend of milk thistle, cayenne pepper, and other herbs. In addition, each capsule contains the following ingredients.

WHITE WILLOW BARK

White willow bark is an aspirinlike herb that contains compounds known as salicylates. They act as pain relievers and antiinflammatories. The herb has been approved by the German Commission E for treating fevers and headaches. Each Cellu-Rid capsule contains 100 milligrams of white willow bark.

POTASSIUM

Potassium is a mineral that, along with sodium, helps regulate fluid balance and distribution in the body. Each capsule of Cellu-Rid is formulated with 20 milligrams of potassium. The recommended daily intake of potassium is 1000 to 1600 milligrams.

IRON

This essential mineral helps create hemoglobin, a protein in your red blood cells that ferries oxygen from the lungs to the rest of your body and is thus vital in healthy circulation. About 73 percent of the iron in your body is found in hemoglobin. If you have an iron deficiency (anemia), not enough hemoglobin is manufactured, and the supply of oxygen to body tissues is reduced. As the saying goes, you have "iron-poor blood" and feel run-down as a result. The recommended intake for men is ten milligrams a day; for women, 15 milligrams a day. Each capsule of Cellu-Rid contains nine milligrams of iron.

COUCH GRASS

A common weed that grows in all fifty states, couch grass is an herbal diuretic that has been used to treat kidney and bladder infections. It helps the body dispose of excess fluid. The German Commission E has approved couch grass for treating urinary and kidney problems. Each capsule of Cellu-Rid is formulated with five milligrams of couch grass.

ASCORBIC ACID (VITAMIN C)

Ascorbic acid, better known as vitamin C, is a water-soluble nutrient that can be synthesized by many animals, but not by humans. It is an essential nutrient in our diets, and functions primarily in the formation of connective tissues such as collagen. Strong, healthy connective tissue helps minimize the appearance of cellulite.

Vitamin C is also involved in immunity, wound healing, and defense against allergies. As an antioxidant, vitamin C keeps free radicals from damaging bodily tissues. There are 80 milligrams of vitamin C in each capsule of Cellu-Rid.

APPLE CIDER VINEGAR

Apple cider vinegar is often found in natural weight loss supplements, usually in partnership with kelp and vitamin B_6, and thought to facilitate fat reduction. Each Cellu-Rid capsule contains 33 milligrams of apple cider vinegar.

GUARANA

Guarana is a red berry from a plant grown in the Amazon Valley. It contains seven times as much caffeine as the coffee bean and is widely sold as a supplement to increase energy. The supplement is made from the seeds of the berry.

Guarana is used in a number of natural weight loss supplements. Its high caffeine content is believed to increase thermogenesis (body heat) and thus stimulate the metabolism. Guarana may also cause your body to release water, since the caffeine it contains is a diuretic. Each Cellu-Rid capsule contains 20 milligrams of guarana.

ROSE HIPS

The dried fruit of roses, rose hips are a rich source of vitamin C and other nutrients. Substances in rose hips help strengthen fragile capillaries and other tissues. There are ten milligrams of rose hips in each capsule of Cellu-Rid.

BUCHU

Derived from the shrub native to South Africa, the leaves of this herb are usually made into a tea and other types of supplements. Buchu is a known diuretic and antiseptic that fights germs in the urinary tract. There are five milligrams of buchu in each Cellu-Rid capsule.

HYDRANGEA

The roots of this plant are used medicinally to treat urinary problems. Each Cellu-Rid capsule is formulated with five milligrams of hydrangea.

HERBACELL PROPRIETARY BLEND

Each Cellu-Rid capsule is formulated with a 200-milligram blend of other herbs. These include senna leaves and cascara sagrada. Both are herbal laxatives that encourage excretion. Also included in the blend are apple extract, milk thistle extract, cayenne pepper, and cinnamon extract.

SUPPLEMENTING WITH CELLU-RID

According to the manufacturer, take one capsule daily, one hour after a meal, with 12 ounces of water. Cellu-Rid costs approximately $25 for a one-month supply. You can order the product from Reach4Life by calling 1–800–214–1814. The herbal doses in Cellu-Rid are considered to be within safe limits by herbalists' standards.

Cellu-Var

Cellu-Var is produced by Enzymatic Therapy, Inc., which manufactures and distributes more than two hundred natural medicines, nutritional supplements, vitamins, and herbal extracts. Cellu-Var is formulated with 30 milligrams of gotu kola extract and ten milligrams of aescin extract from horse chestnut. It also contains 100 milligrams of butcher's broom extract. Butcher's broom is a spiny evergreen shrub that grows in Europe. From its roots and rhizomes (the fleshy, noduled aboveground root of some plants) comes a therapeutic extract containing two antiinflammatory agents, ruscogenin and neoruscogenin, that strengthen veins. The herb has been approved by the German Commission E for treating chronic venous insufficiency and leg cramps.

SUPPLEMENTING WITH CELLU-VAR

According to the manufacturer, you should take one capsule three times daily as an addition to your normal diet. There are sixty capsules in each bottle of Cellu-Var. The product costs $27.45. The herbal doses in Cellu-Var are considered safe by herbalists.

Enzymatic Therapy, Inc., manufactures a companion product called Cellu-Var Cream, which is designed to improve the appearance of cellulitic skin and discolored varicose veins. It contains the herbs rosemary, horse chestnut, and kola nut. One jar costs $12.45.

General Guidelines for Using Herbal Supplements

In the next few years, I believe you are going to see many more anticellulite products on the shelves of pharmacies, grocery stores, and other retailers. That is why it is vital for you to read labels and be able to recognize what the ingredients are and what they do. Because most of the current anticellulite supplements are herb-based, here are some important guidelines to follow if you are thinking about taking herbs as part of your supplement program:

1. Do not take any herbs if you are pregnant or lactating.
2. Educate yourself on herbal therapies and the research, if any, behind them.
3. Purchase herbal supplements from well-known, reputable companies.
4. Look for supplements that are "standardized." This term means the products have been processed to ensure a uniform level of one or more isolated active ingredients from batch to batch. To standardize a product, the manufacturer extracts key active ingredients from the whole herb, measures them, sometimes concentrates them, and then formulates them in a base with other nutrients, including the whole herb. Standardization is a good guarantee of product quality.
5. Read the labels on any herb you might purchase. Make sure you know what each ingredient is and what effect it has on the body. Don't buy the supplement until you've learned all you can about its ingredients and its potential side effects.
6. Some herbs interact dangerously with prescription drugs and should be avoided when you are taking medications. Inform your doctor that you are taking an herbal supplement, especially during an illness or before surgery, or if you have a preexisting medical condition. If you don't communicate this information, you're risking the chance that your doctor may unwittingly prescribe something that will interact dangerously with the supplement. Refer to Table 4.1 for information on some risky combinations.

7. Follow the manufacturer's or doctor's suggestion regarding dosage. Also, pay close attention to any warnings or precautions that appear on the supplement label.
8. Immediately report any adverse effects to your physician.
9. As with medicines, regard all herbs as potentially harmful to children and keep them safely out of reach.

Table 4.1—Potentially Dangerous Herb-Drug Combinations

If you're taking:	Don't combine with:
Antianxiety drugs	*Kava kava
Antibiotics	*St. John's wort
Antidepressants	St. John's wort
Blood thinners	Most cellulite control supplements
Diuretics	Cascara sagrada, senna, or St. John's wort
Laxatives	Cascara sagrada or senna
Sedatives	Kava kava

* Kava kava and St. John's wort are herbs found in herb-based natural weight loss supplements, which are discussed in the next chapter.

CHAPTER 5

Natural Fat Burners

In addition to cellulite control supplements, you may want to consider products known as natural fat burners, particularly if you need to lose body fat. Designed to assist with weight loss and appetite control, natural fat burners are dietary supplements derived or extracted from food or herbs. They exert a much gentler effect on the body than either prescription diet pills or over-the-counter diet drugs do. Best of all, they're effective and easily obtainable.

Natural fat burners are not anticellulite supplements per se, but they can work wonders on overall fat loss when you follow a prudent diet and exercise regularly. Losing body fat minimizes cellulite.

Natural fat burners help ensure that your body has everything it needs to burn fat at peak efficiency. None is a miracle worker, however. If you're overweight, with mild to severe cellulite, and the only change you make in your lifestyle is to take these supplements, nothing will happen, and no cellulite will be erased. For best results, you have to make major improvements in your diet and become more active by exercising regularly. Natural fat burners always work best in combination with a healthy, low-fat diet and a regular exercise program.

Although natural fat burners are generally safe, most of these supplements contain label warnings that should be heeded. If you have concerns about your weight, or suffer from a preexisting illness or medical condition, consult your doctor before taking any of these supplements.

What follows is a look at four broad categories of natural fat burners and how you can use them to your best advantage.

Metabolic Boosters

Failure to lose body fat can be the result of a slow metabolism, possibly brought on by a sluggish thyroid gland. Your thyroid gland controls metabolism—your body's food-to-fuel process. It also secretes hormones that regulate energy, heart rate, body weight, and the use of nutrients. Research shows that supplemental nutrients such as pyruvate, phosphate salts, and guggul may improve thyroid functioning and consequently lead to more efficient fat burning.

Other metabolic boosters include chromium picolinate and conjugated linoleic acid (CLA). These may increase metabolism too, mainly by making more fat available to burn as fuel.

PYRUVATE

Pyruvate, or more specifically pyruvic acid, is made naturally in the body during carbohydrate metabolism and is involved in energy-producing reactions that occur at the cellular level. Pyruvate is also found in tiny amounts in many foods.

The dietary supplements sold as pyruvate are derived from pyruvic acid, which is bonded to a mineral salt, usually calcium, sodium, or potassium. Studied in animals and humans for more than twenty-five years, supplemental pyruvate produces some very desirable metabolic effects in the body, including reduced body fat.

In one study, fifty-three men and women were divided into

one of three groups: a pyruvate group that supplemented with six grams a day of pyruvate for six weeks; a placebo group that supplemented with look-alike pills filled with the carbohydrate maltodextrin; and a control group that received no pills.

All three groups participated in an exercise program thirty minutes a day, three times a week. The pyruvate and placebo groups followed a liberal 2000-calorie-a-day diet.

By the end of the experimental period, the pyruvate-supplemented people had lost 4.6 pounds of body fat, and decreased their body fat percentage by 2.6 percent. By contrast, neither the control group nor the placebo group experienced any significant changes in body fat or percent body fat.

In addition, the pyruvate-supplemented subjects increased their muscle significantly—by 3.3 pounds, on average. Muscle tissue is fat-burning tissue. There were only small gains in lean mass in the other groups.

How exactly does pyruvate work these wonders? Research in both animals and humans shows that pyruvate supplementation elevates the body's resting metabolic rate—probably by increasing levels of thyroxin, a thyroid hormone. Thyroid hormones are chemical regulators of metabolism. Thus, increasing their secretion may boost metabolism.

In addition, researchers believe that pyruvate enhances the oxidation, or burning, of fat. It may also stop the synthesis, or formation, of fat.

How Much to Take

According to available research data, the optimal dose for weight loss is four to six grams a day of pyruvate. For best results, these amounts should be taken in divided doses every four to six hours, preferably with meals. Taking pyruvate throughout the day helps maintain higher levels in your body for more efficient action. As with any natural weight loss supplement, pyruvate does not work for everyone.

Once you reach your fat loss goals, taper down to a maintenance dose of two grams daily for long-term weight control.

PHOSPHATES

Supplementation with phosphates, a type of salt made from the mineral phosphorus, has been scientifically found to increase resting metabolic rate—an action that may confer a fat-burning benefit. Phosphates are one of the ingredients in a supplement called ThyroLean, made by ProLab, which has been specifically formulated to correct a slow-functioning thyroid. Its other ingredients are guggul, an herb; 1-tyrosine, an amino acid that is a building block for thyroid hormones; and hydroxycitric acid, or HCA, the extract of a fruit grown in India. Guggul and HCA can be used individually as natural weight loss supplements (see below).

According to one clinical trial, ThyroLean performed impressively. Over a six-week period, subjects followed an 1800-calorie-a-day diet and exercised three times a week while taking the supplement as recommended.

By the end of the experimental period, the ThyroLean-supplemented subjects had lost 8.3 times as much weight as the controls had lost. That equated to 5.59 pounds, or about .9 pounds a week. In addition, the supplementers lost 45 percent more body fat than the controls lost.

How Much to Take
The manufacturer's recommended dosage of ThyroLean is two capsules three times daily or three capsules twice a day.

GUGGUL

Guggul (*Commiphora mukul*) is an extract purified from the sap, or gummy resin, of a small, thorny tree native to India. It potentially offers an easy, no-willpower way to shed excess weight, and may even restore youthful curves by helping your body incinerate excess fat and calories throughout the day.

In animal studies conducted more than thirty years ago, a scientist in India discovered that test animals lost weight after being given guggul. This sparked interest in guggul as a fat loss agent.

One landmark study conducted in 1990 reported "significant weight loss" in research with seventy guggul-supplemented subjects. Also reported were considerable body composition changes, including less fat under the skin and trimmed-down hip and waist circumferences.

How guggul actually works in this regard is unclear, but scientists speculate that it exerts its effect partially through the activity of the thyroid gland. Guggul appears to spark thyroid activity by increasing levels of the thyroid hormones. When thyroid function is revved up, the body's metabolic rate is increased, leading to more efficient fat-burning.

How Much to Take

To encourage fat loss, informed health practitioners suggest supplementing with one tablet three times a day. Follow the manufacturer's directions for usage, however, since recommended dosages may vary.

CHROMIUM

Chromium is a trace mineral that helps turn carbohydrates into glucose (blood sugar), the fuel burned by cells for energy. Chromium also helps regulate and produce the hormone insulin. Manufactured by the pancreas, insulin helps control hunger, regulates fat storage and muscle-building, and assists the body in utilizing cholesterol properly.

Several studies conducted in the late 1980s and early 1990s found that daily supplements of either 200 or 400 micrograms of chromium picolinate (a form of supplemental chromium) may improve body composition (ratio of fat to muscle) and promote weight loss in healthy adults. One of the very first studies found that supplementing with 200 micrograms of chromium picolinate a day promoted fat loss, *without dieting or exercise*.

In another study, 122 moderately overweight people took either 400 micrograms of chromium picolinate or a placebo daily for several weeks. By the end of the experimental period, the chromium-supplemented volunteers had lost an average of 6.2 pounds of body fat, as opposed to 3.4 pounds in the placebo group.

How exactly does chromium accomplish this? Actually, it's not clear, but there are plausible theories, based on research:

- Chromium may increase the power of insulin to undertake one of its many jobs—producing serotonin, a brain chemical that decreases the appetite.
- Chromium may stimulate the burning of carbohydrates so that they are converted into energy given off as heat, rather than being turned into body fat.
- Chromium may help regulate the body's fat-producing processes. If you eat too many carbohydrates, your body overproduces insulin. Insulin triggers the activity of lipoprotein lipase, an enzyme that tells fat cells to store fat. But, by making insulin work better, chromium, in effect, prevents excess fat from forming.
- Chromium may stimulate the metabolism.
- Chromium aids protein (muscle) synthesis. Assisted by chromium, insulin helps amino acids gain access to cells, where they reassemble themselves to construct new muscle tissue. Thus, chromium may have an indirect effect on muscle growth.

How Much to Take

Chromium researchers who support its use as a weight loss aid recommend taking 200 to 400 micrograms daily, but note that it takes at least eight weeks of supplementation to see results.

CONJUGATED LINOLEIC ACID (CLA)

Discovered in 1978 at the University of Wisconsin, conjugated linoleic acid (CLA) is a naturally occurring fatty acid present in meat, dairy products (particularly cheddar and Colby cheeses), sunflower oil, and safflower oil. It is formed when the bacteria in a cow's gut breaks down linoleic acid in the corn or soybeans the animal eats.

In 1996, CLA became available as a diet product derived from sunflower oil. Ads for CLA note that the nutrient may be missing from many diets (presumably since we tend to eat little meat or high-fat dairy products). The product is promoted as a fat-burning, muscle-toning, energy-boosting agent and is included as a primary ingredient in many weight loss supplements now on health food store shelves. Chromium picolinate is combined with CLA in some products.

No one yet knows how, or if, CLA really exerts a fat-burning effect. Researchers, however, theorize that CLA somehow causes protein, carbohydrates, and fats to be used by cells for energy and muscle tissue growth, rather than stored as fat.

In rat experiments, animals lost half their body fat and gained muscle tissue when fed the human equivalent of one to six grams of CLA daily. In a human study involving CLA, twenty nonobese people (ten men and ten women) were given just over a gram of CLA or a placebo with breakfast, lunch, and dinner. They were instructed not to change their diet or exercise habits.

At the end of three months, the researchers measured both the weight and body fat percentage of the study participants. Even though there was not much difference in weight loss between supplementers and nonsupplementers, there was a huge difference in body fat percentage. The CLA supplementers dropped from 21.3 percent (average body fat) to an average of 17 percent. While it might not sound like much, a reduction of a few points in body fat percentage can make a significant difference in how lean and firm you look. The people taking CLA lost mostly body fat—the ideal situation in any trim-down program.

How Much to Take

Studies of CLA support a dosage of 2.5 to 5 grams a day if you are trying to lose body fat. Follow the manufacturer's recommendations for dosage.

Even though CLA shows tremendous promise, not enough is known yet about it to make a full judgment on its effectiveness. Still, it is worth a try if you're on a cellulite and weight reduction program.

Appetite Suppressants

Want to curb an out-of-control appetite? Try an amino acid formulation containing one or more of the following: dl-phenylalanine, l-tyrosine, l-glutamine, or 5-hydroxy-tryptophan (5-HTP). Taken in supplement form, these substances naturally elevate body chemicals that curb appetite. With your appetite under better control, you're less likely to succumb to food cravings and sudden urges to overeat.

One of the more popular amino acid formulations on the market is a product called PhenCal, which was launched as a natural weight loss aid in June 1997. The manufacturers have tested its effectiveness in two separate studies. In the first one, overweight volunteers supplemented with PhenCal while following a controlled diet and exercise program. They lost an average of 27 pounds in ninety days. Could this weight loss have been due to the other ingredients in PhenCal, such as chromium? Possibly. But the second study sheds more light on why the supplement seems to be effective at promoting weight loss.

This study, which lasted two years, measured PhenCal's effect on food binges among 130 volunteers. Prior to supplementing with PhenCal, the subjects averaged about twelve binges a week. After being treated with PhenCal, they reduced their number of binges by 73 percent (just under four binges a week)—even while following a low-calorie diet and participating in an exercise program. The results of both experiments are quite impressive. The point is that PhenCal may exert its weight loss effect by curbing cravings and keeping a raging appetite at bay. Also, no significant side effects have been reported with PhenCal supplementation. PhenCal, however, does contain phenylalanine, which should be avoided in certain cases (see below).

Another natural appetite suppressant is hydroxycitric acid (HCA), extracted from the Indian fruit *Garcinia cambogia*. When it comes to fat loss, HCA is really a jack-of-all-trades. Not only does it promise to curb your appetite and shut off food cravings, it also appears to block the production of fat, conserve lean muscle, and spare glycogen. That's why you find HCA in so many natural fat burners.

How Much to Take

Natural appetite suppressants come in many different formulations. Follow the manufacturer's recommendations for dosage.

Phenylalanine-containing supplements should be avoided by anyone taking antidepressants; suffering from high blood pressure, the genetic illness phenylketonuria (PKU), diabetes, or migraine headaches; or being treated for melanoma, a serious form of skin cancer. Phenylalanine could aggravate these conditions.

Fat Blockers

In the digestive system, some fibers naturally bind to the fats you eat, trap their molecules, and help escort them from the body. The net effect is to reduce the amount of fat absorbed by the body.

One of these fibers is chitosan. Chitosan is found in at least one cellulite control supplement, CellaFree, discussed in the previous chapter. It has also been combined with HCA and chromium to produce weight loss. In an Italian study, 150 obese subjects were given either the supplement combination or a placebo. Those taking the supplement reduced their weight by 12.5 percent, compared to 4.3 percent among those taking the placebo. Plus, the supplement takers reduced their LDL cholesterol (dubbed "the bad kind") by 35 percent and raised their HDL cholesterol ("the good kind") by 14 percent.

How Much to Take

Depending on the manufacturer's suggestions, you generally take chitosan with water at lunch and dinner. Follow the manufacturer's recommended dosage.

Also, most alternative medicine physicians and nutritionists advise using chitosan for no more than two weeks at a time. This is because it may interfere with the absorption of important nutrients, namely vitamins A, D, E, and K. By blocking their absorption, chitosan could contribute to deficiencies of these essential vitamins. Chitosan products typically state this precaution on their labels.

Herbal Fat Fighters

The cellulite control supplements described in the previous chapter are herb-based formulas. In addition to the herbs in those products, there are others that play a role in weight control. Among the main players are ephedra and *Citrus aurantium.*

From ephedra comes a natural stimulant called ephedrine, shown in scientific research to have powerful thermogenic (heat-producing) and antiobesity properties. Chemically, ephedrine resembles our body's own stimulant, adrenaline (epinephrine), which, among other functions, liberates fat from cells to be used as energy—which is why you find the herb ephedra in many weight loss supplements.

A study conducted in Denmark demonstrated that a supplement made of ephedrine (20 milligrams) and caffeine (200 milligrams) taken three times a day was helpful in promoting weight loss. However, the combination produced central nervous system side effects such as agitation.

I'm not a fan of ephedra, because there are health risks associated with its use, but I do want to mention it because it shows up in so many natural weight loss supplements under various names: ma huang, Chinese ephedra, Mormon tea, Brigham tea, and popotillo. In susceptible individuals, this herb, or its derivative, ephedrine, may produce troublesome side effects, including insomnia, anxiety, nervousness, accelerated heart rate, and high blood pressure.

Further, since 1994, the FDA has received and investigated more than eight hundred complaints of health problems associated with the use of ephedrine-containing products. Among the most serious: heart attacks, stroke, and death. Most occurred in young to middle-aged, otherwise healthy adults using the products for weight control and increased energy. Clearly, there are potentially fatal risks associated with ephedra-containing supplements, so consult your physician before taking them.

Citrus aurantium is the botanical name of the Chinese fruit zhishi. An alkaloid called synephrine is extracted from this fruit and used as an ingredient in numerous fat burners.

Synephrine is a chemical cousin to ephedrine but has few of ephedrine's adverse side effects. Synephrine is thought to suppress the appetite, increase metabolic rate, and help burn fat inside cells. It may prove to be a powerful natural fat fighter, but more research is needed to verify its benefits.

Herbs such as St. John's wort and kava kava are often included in formulations too. Here's why: These herbs have a tranquilizing, uplifting effect on blue moods. Because stress and depression compel many people to overeat, supplementing with either kava kava or St. John's wort may keep you from raiding the fridge in times of trouble.

How Much to Take

Discuss with your physician whether taking herbal fat loss supplements is a good idea. Remember that many herbs interact dangerously with prescription medications. If you get the okay to supplement, follow the recommended dosage on labels of herbal fat loss supplements.

Can You Take Natural Fat Burners with Cellulite Control Supplements?

To date, there is no research data on the merits of taking natural fat burners along with cellulite-control supplements. Until more is known, it is wise to supplement with one *or* the other. For example, you might take a cellulite control supplement for eight to twelve weeks only, then afterward try a natural fat burner if you need assistance in your fat loss efforts.

Many natural fat burners can be used concurrently. For example, pyruvate and chromium are often taken together, and some products contain formulations of the two.

However, be careful about taking a handful of different products at the same time. It's unclear how well some combinations work. They may enhance the effects of one another; they may not.

To reiterate, it's better to try one supplement or one product at a time. Then give each supplement several weeks before deciding whether it's helping you lose weight. If you stop seeing results from one that works, cycle it; that is, go on and off the supplement. Take it for a couple weeks at a time, discontinue it, and then resume supplementation. Remember too that what works for someone else may not work as well for you. Each of us is quite different in how our bodies respond to various nutrients.

CHAPTER 6

Nutritional Support Supplements

Nutritional supplementation holds an important place in treating, minimizing, and preventing cellulite. It provides extra insurance that you are giving your body all the resources it needs to become cellulite resistant. Supplementation, however, works hand in hand with good nutrition. While supplementing, you should be following a nutritious diet, such as the one outlined in the 30-Day Anticellulite Diet in chapter 8.

What follows is a look at the several nutritional support supplements you might consider taking as part of a comprehensive program against cellulite.

Antioxidants

Some medical experts believe that free radicals contribute to the development of cellulite. Mentioned elsewhere in this book, free radicals are unstable oxygen molecules that attack bodily tissues, including blood vessels. The damage they do results in inflammation and abnormal drainage of blood and lymph into surrounding tissues.

Many factors give rise to these biological terrorists, including normal metabolism, aging, stress, sunlight, and exposure to environmental toxins such as cigarette smoke, exhaust fumes, and other pollutants.

Fortunately though, your body is equipped with a mighty defense team of substances known as antioxidants that squelch free radicals and prevent them from doing harm. Vitamin C, vitamin E, and beta-carotene are the chief vitamin antioxidants. The antioxidant minerals include selenium, zinc, copper, and manganese. They're involved synergistically in the formation and activity of antioxidant enzymes, agents that inactivate free radicals.

A chief collagen-strengthening nutrient, vitamin C keeps free radicals from destroying the outermost layers of cells and has the power to regenerate vitamin E. Vitamin C also helps promote the health of your blood vessels.

Known as one of nature's most effective antioxidants, vitamin E prevents a free radical–initiated process known as lipid peroxidation. In a dominolike series of chemical reactions, free radicals hook up with fatty acids in the body to form substances called peroxides. Peroxides attack cell membranes, setting off a chain reaction that creates many more free radicals. Pits form in cell membranes, allowing harmful bacteria, viruses, and other disease-causing agents to gain entry into cells.

Vitamin E also protects beta-carotene from destruction in the body and is an important guardian of blood vessel health. In addition, emerging research suggests that vitamin E may safeguard the skin against wrinkling.

Beta-carotene is a member of a group of substances known as carotenoids. There are more than four hundred carotenoids in nature, found mostly in orange and yellow fruits and vegetables, and in dark green vegetables.

Once ingested, beta-carotene is converted to vitamin A in the body on an as-needed basis. As an antioxidant, beta-carotene's main role is to detoxify a highly energetic, free radical–like product called singlet oxygen. Like a server in a cafeteria line, singlet oxygen dishes out its energy to hungry molecules in the line. This process generates many more free radicals. Beta-carotene comes along, shuts the line down by absorbing the singlet oxygen's energy, and puts it out of commission. This amazing nutrient can also destroy free radicals after they're formed.

Antioxidant minerals work by supplying the elements your body needs to make antioxidant enzymes. Selenium, for example, produces glutathione peroxidase, an antioxidant enzyme that can turn troublesome free radicals into harmless water. On its own, selenium has other antioxidant functions. It appears to preserve the elasticity of tissues by delaying the free radical–induced destruction of fatty acids. This mineral also works closely with vitamin E in protecting the body against free radicals. Selenium deficiencies have been associated with premature aging.

Copper, zinc, and manganese work as antioxidants too. All three help make superoxide dismutase (SOD), an antioxidant enzyme that neutralizes certain types of free radicals.

To ensure sufficient antioxidant intake and protection from free radicals, it is wise to take a once-a-day vitamin/mineral tablet containing antioxidant nutrients. You may also want to consider supplementing with more vitamin C and vitamin E than can be found in a multiple vitamin/mineral supplement.

Choose a natural form of vitamin E over a synthetic version. Labeled as d-alpha tocopherol, natural vitamin E is isolated from soybean, sunflower, corn, peanut, grape seed, and cottonseed oils. Synthetic vitamin E, or dl-alpha tocopherol, is processed from substances found in petrochemicals. A recent review of thirty published studies on vitamin E concluded that the natural version is absorbed better by the body than the synthetic form.

Based on available evidence on antioxidants, here are suggested daily intakes:

- 10,000 to 20,000 International Units of beta carotene
- 400 to 800 International Units of vitamin E

- 200 to 500 milligrams of vitamin C
- Up to 50 micrograms of selenium
- Two milligrams of copper
- 12 milligrams of zinc
- Up to five milligrams of manganese

Calcium

What's good for your bones may also be good for your skin. That's a recent hypothesis put forward by research scientists working in the field of dermatology. They base their assumption on the medical fact that both skin and bone are composed of more than 70 percent of the same type of collagen. So if you protect bone health through calcium supplementation, exercise, and other healthy practices, quite possibly you could be slowing down the aging of your skin at the same time.

It will be interesting to see how this hypothesis shakes out in the future. But for now, taking calcium supplements and exercising are important for another reason that has an indirect bearing on the treatment and elimination of cellulite: They protect you from osteoporosis, a crippling age-related loss of bone that can keep you from living an active life and building a cellulite-resistant body.

On average, everyone starts losing bone around age thirty-five, but the loss speeds up in women after menopause. For women, supplementing with calcium and exercising offer an extra measure of protection. So says evidence from a number of studies, including one from Australia. There, researchers studied three treatments for osteoporosis to determine which worked the best—exercise only, exercise plus calcium, or exercise plus estrogen.

After all the data was compiled on the 120 postmenopausal women who participated, it turned out that both the exercise-plus-calcium treatment and the exercise-plus-estrogen treatment slowed or prevented bone loss. The exercise-estrogen treatment was more effective, however. But the women in that group experienced unpleasant side effects, such as breast tenderness and vaginal bleeding. What this study hints at is that there's a natural way to treat bone loss—exercise and calcium supplementation—without having to resort to prescription medication.

I'm sure you want to be physically active for as long as possible—in order to control your weight, minimize cellulite, and stay fit. Accordingly, you have to pull out all the stops to ensure lifelong health and vitality. As the research shows, one of the best ways to do that is by getting enough calcium and staying active.

For women, the current recommendations for calcium are 1200 milligrams daily before menopause and 1500 milligrams daily after menopause. Dependable sources of calcium, in addition to supplements, include low-fat dairy products, calcium-fortified fruit juices, and green leafy vegetables.

Fiber Supplements

Constipation aggravates cellulite by causing water retention, preventing normal excretion of waste products, and interfering with the proper lymphatic drainage in the legs. The 30-Day Anticellulite Diet in chapter 8 is high in fiber and should help counter constipation. But if your digestive system is particularly stubborn, you may want to take a natural fiber supplement each day. Supplementing with fiber is also an excellent weight-control measure.

Case in point: Mildly obese women who ate a six- or seven-gram fiber supplement while following a 1200-to-1600-calorie-a-day diet lost significantly more weight (about six pounds) in eleven weeks than the placebo takers did, plus were able to stick to their diets better.

Most fiber supplements contain either psyllium or citrus pectin as their active high-fiber ingredient. Psyllium is a natural, bulk-forming substance made from the seeds of the plantago plant, cultivated in Europe. Found in supplements such as

Metamucil, psyllium is known for its ability to hold water and form a gel in the stomach. This adds bulk and can make you feel full.

Psyllium is a gentle, effective agent that passes through the intestinal tract, holding fluids, toxins, and other waste products as it goes. The extra bulk it provides enhances elimination. Its bulk-forming ability may help curb your desire to eat. Also, research has found that psyllium ushers undigested fat from the body.

Some people may be allergic to psyllium. Reactions can range from a mild rash to breathing problems, even death. It may also interfere with the absorption of some vitamins and minerals, so don't take a psyllium supplement at the same time as you take a vitamin/mineral pill or a cellulite control supplement. Be sure to take psyllium with at least eight ounces of water to prevent possible obstructions in the esophagus or stomach.

Citrus pectin is another agent found in many fiber supplements. Derived from citrus fruits, it is a water-soluble fiber that provides gentle relief from constipation. Citrus pectin has a cholesterol-lowering effect too. By binding to bile acids (a source of cholesterol in the body) in the intestines, pectin keeps cholesterol from recycling, thus reducing the body's total cholesterol pool. Like psyllium, it escorts fat from the body too.

An inexpensive, effective way to supplement with fiber is to sprinkle one or two tablespoons of wheat bran on your cereal each morning. Bran is one of several high-fiber foods that not only prevents constipation, but also binds to some of the fat you eat and escorts it from the body. Other foods with the same benefits included whole wheat products and rolled oats.

When using fiber supplements, do not exceed the manufacturer's suggested daily dose. Overdosing on fiber supplements flushes vital nutrients from the body and may lead to dependency on the supplement. Abusing any type of fiber supplement can damage the nerves responsible for the colonic contractions that move waste products out of the body.

Energy Bars and Drinks

The 30-Day Anticellulite Diet recommends snacking occasionally on energy bars for a nutritious midmorning or midafternoon pick-me-up. Wildly popular and available at gyms, health food stores, and grocery stores, these candy bar–like products are specially formulated with protein, carbohydrates, fats, and other nutrients. As for calories, the range is wide. Some bars have as few as 130 calories; others go as high as 500 calories.

The problem with many bars, however, is that they are as high in fat and simple sugars as a standard candy bar— definitely not what you need when trying to get lean and firm. Fat and sugar can derail your efforts to build a cellulite-resistant body.

The key is to find a bar that is low in sugar and fat. If the first few ingredients listed on the label read sucrose, dextrose, fructose, or any word ending in "ose," that particular energy bar is probably too high in sugar.

Fructose, in fact, is the worst possible sugar to consume on a fat loss diet. In the body, fructose can be fat-forming. Although it is a natural sugar found in fruit, fructose has a different molecular structure than other sugars and, consequently, your body uses it differently. During digestion, fructose bypasses a certain control point that decides if a dietary sugar is going to be stored as energy in the form of glycogen or deposited as fat. Most other natural carbohydrates such as rice, whole grains, and potatoes are preferentially stored as glycogen. But if not used first as energy, fructose is directly converted to fat in the liver. It is then whisked off to the bloodstream to be stored in fat cells.

The bar I recommend for fat loss diets is the Parrillo Energy Bar, manufactured by Parrillo Performance of Cincinnati, Ohio. It is one of the few low-sugar, low-fat energy bars on the market. Each bar contains 14 grams of protein, 35 grams of healthy carbohydrates (oat bran, rice bran, and brown rice), less than one gram of conventional fat, and only three grams of sugar. There are 230 calories in each bar. The product comes in five flavors: French Vanilla, Sweet Milk Chocolate, Apple Cinnamon, Chocolate Raspberry, and Butter Rum.

The main sweetening agent in these energy bars is a newly approved sweetener called Sucralose. It is six hundred times sweeter than table sugar, and remarkably it is made from a process that begins with regular sugar.

Sucralose is slowly finding its way into more and more foods. It has been approved for use in many products, including baked goods, baking mixes, nonalcoholic beverages, chewing gum, desserts, fruit juices, confections, toppings, and syrups, among many others. You can bake with it, and it can be added directly to foods.

The Parrillo Energy Bar can be ordered by calling 1–800–344–3404. For more information on the product, call 1–513–531–1311, or visit the manufacturer's Web site at www.parrillo.com.

Another excellent snack on the 30-Day Anticellulite Diet is an energy drink or meal replacer, available in cans, or mix-it-yourself powders. They are formulated to reproduce as closely as possible the nutrition you would get from food, complete with carbohydrates, protein, fat, vitamins, and minerals.

You can buy meal replacers in health food stores, gyms, sporting goods stores, pharmacies, and grocery stores. The canned versions are a bit pricey—up to two dollars a serving. You can save money by using the powder form, although the powders take more time to fix.

As with energy bars, select products that are low in sugar and fat. Read labels carefully.

Meal replacers should be used only as a supplement to your diet, not as a substitute for meals. The best way to fuel your body is always by eating a nutrient-dense diet of a variety of low-fat proteins and dairy products, fruits, grains, vegetables, and legumes.

88

Purchasing Quality Supplements

Nutritional supplements are not regulated or approved by the FDA as prescription drugs are—so it's hard to know whether you're buying a quality product. A good rule of thumb is to try to find brands from well-known manufacturers such as pharmaceutical companies. Finally, if you choose to supplement, follow the manufacturer's recommendation for dosage and always get your doctor's approval before supplementing.

PART III

Anticellulite Nutrition

CHAPTER 7

Nutritional Cellulite Busters

Minimizing cellulite calls for attacking it on all fronts, including diet. Used in conjunction with supplementation and exercise, the right foods can work wonders in firming up your figure and helping you iron out cellulite. Anticellulite nutrition:

- supplies the nutrients your skin needs to strengthen and reinforce its underlying dermal structures and connective tissue.
- provides nutritional building blocks for the construction of body-firming muscle.
- encourages more efficient fat-burning.
- regulates water balance and fights water retention.
- energizes your body to perform anticellulite exercises. You'll have more energy all day long because you'll be fueling your body with high-grade food.
- helps you look great in leg-baring outfits.

There are ten elements of a successful anticellulite nutrition program, described in the following pages and integrated into my 30-Day Anticellulite Diet in the next chapter. See if you can incorporate the following cellulite busters into your diet to whittle away fat and smooth out cellulite—and do it healthfully.

Cellulite Buster #1: Eat Protein-Rich Foods

Found in every cell in your body, protein is a growth and maintenance nutrient. You get protein primarily from animal foods, although it is also found in many vegetables such as soybeans and other legumes. Protein is made up of nitrogen-containing units called amino acids, which are reshuffled back into protein to make and repair body tissues.

Protein is critical to fat-burning in two important ways. First, high-protein meals can elevate your metabolism by as much as 30 percent above normal for up to twelve hours, compared to about 4 percent for a carbohydrate meal. With ample protein in your diet, your metabolism runs in high gear to burn more fat.

Second, protein is involved in building the most metabolically active tissue in your body—muscle. Daily activity, including exercise, causes a natural breakdown of muscle tissue. For muscle tissue to build itself back up and form new tissue, your body needs protein for growth and repair.

If you don't get enough protein and you're active, your body can start breaking down muscle tissue to get amino acids for energy. Consequently, you'll lose lean muscle and derail your fat loss efforts.

The more muscle you develop through a protein-rich diet and proper exercise, the more efficient your body becomes at burning fat. Adding just one pound of muscle to your body helps you burn an additional 18,000 to 25,000 calories a year.

Protein has another talent: Together with certain minerals, it helps regulate the proper amount of water in areas of the body. This happens because proteins are hydrophilic, or attractive to water. Water molecules thus tend to congregate near the proteins.

When your diet is protein deficient, proteins in the blood become depleted. Without enough protein to cling to, water in the vascular spaces leaks out into the spaces between the cells. Once there, it cannot be excreted by the kidneys, and the result is edema, or water retention.

In short, protein is vital to a speedy metabolism; it helps build new tissue, including muscle and connective tissue, and it is involved in regulating water balance. For these reasons, protein is truly a powerful anticellulite nutrient.

The best protein choices include the following:

- egg whites, cooked
- fish (any type)
- nonfat yogurt and other low-fat dairy products
- shellfish
- soybeans
- sugar-free protein powders and supplements
- sugar-free soy milk
- white-meat chicken
- white-meat turkey

Where fat loss is concerned, some of the current thinking indicates that a daily protein intake of between 25 and 30 percent of daily calories is needed to maintain muscle while losing fat. I agree with that recommendation, since better muscle firmness and shape can be achieved with a moderately high amount of protein in the diet. The 30-Day Anticellulite Diet in the next chapter contains protein-rich daily menus.

Here's how to figure your protein needs for a 1200-calorie diet:

- Multiply protein needs by 25 percent: **1200 × .25 = 300 calories from protein.**
- Divide 300 by 4, since there are 4 calories in a gram of protein: **300 ÷ 4 = 75 grams of protein a day.**
- Divide 75 grams by 3 for at least three meals that include protein (breakfast, lunch, and dinner, although you could have protein with snacks too for a total of five meals): **75 ÷ 3 = 25 grams of protein per meal or snack.**

To help you plan, there are about 25 grams of protein in three ounces of white meat poultry, fish, and lean meat; eight grams in a cup of skim milk or nonfat yogurt; 18 grams in a four-ounce serving of tofu, and about eight grams in a half cup of cooked beans or legumes. If you don't like to fuss with gram counting, just have a few ounces of protein with each meal, and you'll easily satisfy your protein requirement.

Cellulite Buster #2: Slash Your Fat Intake

Fatty foods can quickly derail your attempts to firm up. The main reason: Calories from fat (butter, fried foods, cheeses, candy, and so forth) are readily stored as body fat, whereas calories from other foods have to be converted to fat—a process that burns calories.

An easy way to raise your fat-burning potential is to slash the fat in your diet. Sometimes that's all you need to do to reduce calories. In one study, a group of women ate as much as they wanted, but stuck to low-fat versions of their favorite foods. This low-fat fare automatically cut 220 calories a day from their diets, and the women lost an average of a half pound a week.

Reduce your intake of high-fat foods by sticking to low-fat and nonfat choices: lean proteins like white-meat poultry, fish, and egg whites, low-fat dairy products, low-fat salad dressings, and other reduced-fat foods.

In addition, learn how to cut the fat from your diet by making healthful substitutions. For example: a baked potato for french fries; skim milk for whole milk, plain yogurt for sour cream or mayonnaise, ice milk or frozen yogurt for ice cream, a grilled chicken sandwich for a cheeseburger, fat-free pretzels for potato chips, to name just a few lower-fat substitutions. Also, broil, bake, or microwave foods rather than frying them.

Watch out for "hidden" fat in certain foods too. Fat is added to crackers, cookies, breads, and rolls. You may not see it, but it's there.

Also important: You need some dietary fat for energy and good health, but how much?

There's some disparity in the scientific community as to how much total fat you should eat daily. Many dietitians and health associations recommend that total fat calories should represent less than 30 percent of your total calories. This is a healthy, safe recommendation.

Every person is different, however, since no two metabolisms are exactly alike. Twenty percent of total calories from fat may work perfectly for one person, but not another. You really must find out for yourself. Remember though, you do need some dietary fat for energy. Also, fat keeps your joints, skin, and internal organs in good working order. The daily fat intake in the 30-Day Anticellulite Diet ranges from 10 to 30 percent of total calories.

The following list includes the healthiest fats you can eat. Limit yourself to no more than one tablespoon daily.

- canola oil
- flaxseed oil
- olive oil
- safflower oil
- soybean oil
- sunflower seed oil

Cellulite Buster #3: Fill Up on Fiber

There's an incredibly easy, no-willpower way to manage your weight—one that most of us should be doing but aren't: eating more fiber. More fiber in your diet will help transform your dieting efforts into something simple and automatic. You'll be able to keep your weight under control, without even working at it or making yourself crazy.

Fiber (also called "roughage") is the nondigestible portion of plant foods. There are two types, soluble and insoluble. Soluble fiber turns into a gel when mixed with water. Good sources include rice, corn, oats, legumes, citrus fruits, bananas, carrots, prunes, and seeds. Insoluble fiber absorbs water like a sponge. Examples of foods rich in insoluble fiber include root and leafy vegetables, whole grains, and legumes. Apples, pears, and berries are excellent sources of both soluble and insoluble fiber.

It's really amazing what a little extra fiber can do. Researchers at the University of Kentucky asked people to consume high-fiber oat bran muffins or cooked beans in their diets—without making any other dietary changes. The simple addition of extra fiber resulted in 2.2 pounds lost over a three-week period—automatically and without dieting.

A diet high in fiber will help keep you firm and lean—for several reasons:

- Fiber makes you feel full. Numerous studies have found that eating more fiber or taking a fiber supplement curbs hunger.
- More energy (calories) is spent digesting and absorbing high-fiber foods.
- Fiber lowers insulin levels (insulin is a hormone that stimulates fat production).
- Fiber reduces hunger by stimulating the release of appetite-suppressing hormones.
- Fiber increases the time it takes for food to move through your system, meaning fewer calories are left to be stored as fat.

To get the protective benefits from fiber, the National Research Council recommends eating 20 to 35 grams of fiber a day. As I pointed out in the previous chapter, you may want to take a fiber supplement each day to ensure that you get enough fiber in your diet.

Cellulite Buster #4:
Moderate Your Intake of Carbohydrates

Carbohydrates include such foods as cereals, whole grains, breads, pasta, rice, potatoes, yams, legumes, vegetables, and

Table 7.1—Healthy Sources of Carbohydrates

High-Starch Carbohydrates	Low-Starch Carbohydrates	Fruits
• Barley	Alfalfa sprouts	Blackberries
• Beans	Asparagus	Blueberries
- Black beans	Bamboo shoots	Boysenberries
- Broadbeans	Beans, green	Cantaloupe
- Garbanzo beans	Beans, yellow or wax	Cherries
- Great Northern	Beans, French cut	Cranberries
- Kidney beans	Beet greens	Dried fruits
- Lima beans	Broccoflower	Granny Smith
- Pinto beans	Broccoli	apples
- Red beans	Broccoli sprouts	Grapes
- Snap beans	Brussels sprouts	Green pears
- Soybeans	Cabbage, all varieties	Honeydew melon
- White beans	Carrots	Kiwifruit
• Beets	Cauliflower	Peaches
• Black-eyed peas	Celery	Pineapple
• Bran	Collard greens	Raspberries, black
• Bulgur wheat	Cucumbers	Strawberries
• Corn, sweet	Eggplant	Watermelon
• Corn grits	Endive	
• Corn tortillas (unfried)	Kale	
• Cream of Wheat	Leeks	
• Kasha	Lettuce, all varieties	
• Lentils	Mushrooms	
• Parsnips	Mustard greens	
• Peas	Onions	
• Popcorn, oil-free, air-popped	Peppers, green, red, yellow	
• Potatoes	Peppers, hot	
• Pumpkin	Pimientos	
• Rice, brown	Radishes	
• Rice, puffed	Spinach	
• Shredded wheat	Summer squash, all varieties	
• Rutabagas		
• Sweet potatoes	Tomato juice	
• Wheat germ	Tomatoes	
• Winter squash	Turnips	
• Yams	Turnip greens	
	Vegetable juice	
	Watercress	
	Zucchini	

fruits. As energy foods, carbohydrates are absolutely essential, and must be included in your diet. But if you want to speed up your fat loss, curtail your carbohydrate intake slightly. When you reduce carbohydrates, your body has less glycogen (stored sugar) to run on, so it starts burning more fat instead.

Include a natural, high-starch carbohydrate such as cereal, rice, or potatoes at every meal except dinner. That way, you'll still have enough carbohydrates earlier in the day when you need them the most for exercise and other activities. If you can stand it, eliminate high-starch carbohydrates altogether after midafternoon. Cutting these out in the evening reduces the number of calories at dinner. That's good—since a light evening meal is better for fat loss. Save your bigger meals for breakfast and lunch.

The categories of carbohydrates to include in your diet are listed in Table 7.1.

Generally speaking, your daily carbohydrate intake for fat loss should be around 50 percent of your total caloric intake. Here's how to figure your carbohydrate needs on a 1200-calorie-a-day diet:

- Multiply calorie needs by 50 percent: **1200 × .50 = 600 calories from carbohydrates.**
- Divide 600 by 4, since there are 4 calories in a gram of carbohydrate: **600 ÷ 4 = 150 grams of carbohydrate a day.**
- Divide 150 grams by 4 for breakfast, midmorning snack, lunch, and midafternoon snack: **140 ÷ 4 = 37.5 grams of carbohydrate per meal or snack.**

Usually, you'll consume the amount you need by including a half cup to a full cup of vegetables or grains, or a piece of fruit at each major meal—without having to do any calculations. What's more, the 30-Day Anticellulite Diet does all your nutrient calculations for you.

Keep in mind that everyone is different. You may need fewer (or more) carbohydrates than the formula states. Let your energy level be your guide.

Cellulite Buster #5: Reduce Your Intake of Sugar

Sugars—honey, syrup, table sugar, brown sugar—are quickly digested into glucose, a sugar in the blood that is converted into glycogen for the muscles and liver or carried in the blood to fuel the brain and muscles. If you eat too much sugar at once, the excess can be turned into body fat. This happens because excess sugar triggers a surge of the hormone insulin. Insulin activates certain enzymes that promote fat storage. Natural complex carbohydrates don't cause this reaction—which is why they're less likely to be stored as fat.

There's another bit of bad news regarding sugar: An excess of sugary foods can suppress blood flow to fatty tissue. Reduced blood flow prevents fat from being burned. So avoid excess sugar if you're fighting fat and cellulite.

Sugar is your enemy if you want to stay fit and cellulite resistant, but did you know that it may speed up the age-related changes in collagen—the major constituent of connective tissue? Research suggests that sugar rushing into the bloodstream as glucose starts a reaction that causes proteins (including collagen) in cell membranes to cross-link, an undesirable process in which protein molecules become chemically bound to each other. Cross-linking leads to a loss of elasticity in the skin, and is thought to be a major factor in the aging process. Quite possibly, by limiting sugar in your diet you can prevent further age-related collagen degradation.

Cellulite Buster #6: Consume Naturally Diuretic Foods

Water retention masquerades as pudge and is thought to aggravate cellulite. Let's say you weigh 150 pounds. About 90 of those pounds are water; 30 are fat. The rest is lean tissue—muscles, organs, and bones. So normally, most of your body weight is water. Sometimes you may retain water. You look and feel "fat," even though you may have lost a significant amount of body fat. Some days, you can't even fit into clothes you wore the week before!

That's why it's important to prevent tissues from becoming waterlogged. A natural way to fight bloat is by populating your diet with foods thought to be diuretic, meaning they help the body eliminate water.

Most high-diuretic foods fall into the fruit and vegetable category. Some of the best include:

- alfalfa sprouts
- apples
- asparagus
- beets
- cherries
- cranberries
- cucumbers
- grapes
- onions
- parsley
- pineapple
- strawberries
- watercress
- watermelon

The therapeutic action of these foods depends largely on their mineral content. They happen to be very high in potassium, which promotes proper disposal of the body's wastes, and phosphorus, which helps maintain kidney functioning. Both minerals help regulate the fluid balance in your body.

It's also worth mentioning that in addition to their diuretic qualities, these fruits and vegetables are teeming with other nutrients and should become constants in your regular diet. Try to eat two to three servings from this list daily.

Other naturally diuretic nutrients are herbs, and most are a gentle, nontoxic way to rid your body of excess fluids.

The most effective herbal diuretics are fennel, alfalfa, parsley, chamomile, rose hips, and uva ursi. You can obtain these herbs in easy-to-take capsules or delicious herbal teas. Several supplement companies manufacture special herbal diuretic preparations made from combinations of these herbs. Some of these herbs are included in cellulite control supplements.

Your favorite health food store should have a plentiful supply of health-giving herbal remedies. Always follow the manufacturer's recommended dosage and report any untoward reactions to your physician.

A vitamin that appears to fight bloat safely is B_6 (pyridoxine). Medical experts, however, caution against dosages over 200 milligrams a day without medical supervision. Research has shown that huge dosages of B_6 can be extremely toxic.

Cellulite Buster #7: Eat Foods High in Vitamin C

For minimizing cellulite, vitamin C is an important nutrient because of its involvement in the growth and development of connective tissue, particularly collagen. Firm, healthy connective tissue helps reduce the appearance of cellulite.

Interestingly, in test tubes, vitamin C triggers the manufacture of collagen. Without vitamin C, the body produces abnormal, faulty collagen, and the result is a disease called scurvy. Its symptoms include bleeding gums, fragile skin, easy bleeding and bruising, poor wound healing, and loss of bone and teeth. Outbreaks of scurvy in the 1800s claimed the lives of many British sailors until it was discovered that eating citrus fruits could prevent it. Lime juice was then put on all British sailing ships, and British sailors were nicknamed "limeys." Today, scurvy is rare in the United States.

Vitamin C is also involved in immunity, wound healing, and allergic responses. As an antioxidant, vitamin C protects cells from free radical damage. It also has diuretic properties.

The best sources of vitamin C are citrus fruits. Other foods, such as green and red peppers, collard greens, broccoli, brussels sprouts, cabbage, spinach, potatoes, cantaloupe, and strawberries are also excellent sources too. Try to eat at least two high-vitamin-C foods a day. Supplementing with 500 milligrams a day is good insurance against deficiencies.

Foods rich in vitamin C are also high in nutrients called bioflavonoids, also known as vitamin P. Found in practically all plant foods, bioflavonoids work together with vitamin C to maintain healthy collagen. In fact, one of the principal functions of bioflavonoids is keeping collagen strong and resistant to inflammation. They also strengthen capillaries.

Cellulite Buster #8: Eat Multiple Meals

Gone are the days of three squares only! Which is probably good news, since most people like to nibble throughout the day anyway. Eating frequently throughout the day has several fat-burning and nutritional advantages:

- **A higher calorie-burn rate.** Every time you eat a meal, your metabolic rate goes up as heat is given off to digest and absorb food. By eating five meals a day, your metabolism has extra opportunities to stay cranked up, and that means more fat-burning power.
- **More energy.** With frequent meals, your body has a constant stream of energy-giving nutrients. When it's time to exercise, you'll be full of pep and ready to go.
- **Better absorption of nutrients.** Eating smaller, more frequent meals helps your body better use vitamins and minerals. Research has shown that a higher percentage of nutrients are absorbed with a series of small meals, compared to two or three large ones.
- **Less temptation** to stray from your fat-losing nutritional program. When you're eating five times a day, every two or three hours, you're less likely to binge on foods you shouldn't

have. Nor do you get hungry or prone to cravings. In short, frequent meals shore up your willpower.

A final tip: Don't skip breakfast! If you do, you'll burn about 5 percent fewer calories than people who start the day with a meal. Eating breakfast also helps control hunger pangs through the rest of the day.

Cellulite Buster #9: Limit Your Alcohol Consumption

Alcoholic beverages are loaded with sugary calories (and sugar is easily converted into body fat) and low in nutritional value. Plus, when there's alcohol in your system, the liver works overtime to process it and doesn't have adequate time to burn fat. A study conducted at the University of Lausanne, in Switzerland, found that the addition of pure alcohol (three ounces a day) to the diet resulted in about one-third less fat being burned. Clearly, drinking alcohol subtracts from your body's fat-burning power.

Not only that, excessive alcohol use leads to water retention and increases your chances of developing heart disease, high blood pressure, liver disease, certain cancers, and nutritional deficiencies, among other health-threatening conditions.

Cellulite Buster #10: Drink Plenty of Water

Water is important from a fat-burning perspective. The kidneys need ample water to do their job of filtering waste products from the body. If water is in short supply, the kidneys can't filter properly, so they turn to the liver for help. One of the liver's many responsibilities is mobilizing stored fat for energy. But when it takes over for the kidneys, the liver can't do its fat-burning job as well. This can hinder fat loss.

The amount of water you need daily depends on your weight. Generally, an average adult needs approximately eight to ten eight-ounce glasses of water a day to maintain a healthy water balance.

There's an easy way to tell whether or not you've had enough water: Check the color of your urine. Clear-colored urine indicates that you are well hydrated; dark-colored urine means you are dehydrated. The reason for the dark color is an accumulation of metabolic waste not adequately filtered.

Try to drink water throughout the day. Because you'll be exercising, a good rule of thumb is: Drink a glass or two before you exercise, sip water during exercise, and then have another glass or two after exercise.

Getting Results

It's not possible to predict fat loss or cellulite reduction precisely, even for people following the exact same eating plan. Results vary from person to person, depending on the stage of cellulite formation, activity level, motivation, present physical condition, and percentage of body fat and lean muscle upon starting the program. Nevertheless, everyone who follows these nutritional strategies to the letter will see some results.

On average, you should be able to lose between one and two pounds of body fat a week. That's the safest rate of weight loss as recommended by medical professionals.

If You Don't Need to Lose Body Fat . . .

But still want to smooth out cellulite, follow my suggested cellulite busters, with these modifications:

- Eat more food (over and above the 1200 calories a day). Begin to gradually increase your calories every few days until you reach 2000 or 2500 calories.
- Modify your diet so that 65 to 75 percent of your total daily calories come from natural carbohydrates. There's a reason for this: You're probably a fast metabolizer, which means your body burns up food as fast as you consume it. Research

has found that fast metabolizers do well on a diet that's higher in carbohydrates—unlike slow metabolizers, who do better on fewer carbohydrates.

- Make sure you're eating three large meals a day, with two or three smaller, snack-type meals in between.

CHAPTER 8

The 30-Day Anticellulite Diet

Featuring thirty days of menus, the 30-Day Anticellulite Diet* incorporates many of the cellulite busters described in chapter 7. It is not a rigid diet, but rather a general guide for how to eat each day. You may want to follow this plan exactly as written, or adapt it to your own food preferences.

On average, the plan provides approximately 1000 to 1200 calories a day; usually no more than 25 percent of those calories come from fat. If you are very active and work out religiously five or six times a week, you may want to increase calories—to 1500 or more daily. This can be accomplished by eating larger servings of grains and breads, vegetables, and fruits.

This plan is also moderately high in protein, while providing moderate amounts of carbohydrates—two dietary strategies that encourage fat loss. It includes naturally diuretic foods, vitamin C–rich foods, and fiber.

Eat well, and enjoy!

* Nutrients in the 30-Day Anticellulite Diet Plan were analyzed using Diet Expert software.

DAY 1

BREAKFAST
  ½ cup Raisin Bran
  1 cup skim milk
  1 cup fresh strawberries (or other seasonal fruit)
  1 cup herbal tea

MIDMORNING SNACK
  1 granola bar

LUNCH
  3 ounces water-packed tuna with one sliced tomato served
    on a generous bed of lettuce
  2 tablespoons low-fat Italian dressing

MIDAFTERNOON SNACK
  1 cup nonfat plain yogurt mixed with 1 tablespoon low-
    calorie strawberry preserves

DINNER
  5 ounces roasted chicken breast
  1 cup cooked asparagus spears
  1 cup cubed watermelon

Daily Nutrition Profile: *1031 calories, 39 percent protein, 41
percent carbohydrate, 20 percent fat, 184 milligrams vitamin C,
and 15 grams dietary fiber.*

DAY 2

BREAKFAST
  3 scrambled egg whites
  1 oat bran muffin
  ½ grapefruit
  1 cup herbal tea

MIDMORNING SNACK
    2 low-sodium rice cakes
    1 ounce fat-free American cheese

LUNCH
    Quick fajitas: 1 cup cooked black beans, 2 flour tortillas,
        2 tablespoons salsa, 2 tablespoons chopped fresh onion

MIDAFTERNOON SNACK
    1 cup melon balls

DINNER
    5 ounces grilled salmon
    1 cup cooked broccoli
    1 cup cooked carrots

*Daily Nutrition Profile: 1195 calories; 29 percent protein, 56
percent carbohydrate, 15 percent fat, 184 milligrams vitamin C,
and 28 grams dietary fiber.*

DAY 3

BREAKFAST
    1 ounce granola cereal mixed into 1 cup nonfat plain
        yogurt
    1 cup cranberry juice
    1 cup herbal tea

MIDMORNING SNACK
    1 medium apple

LUNCH
    Mediterranean sandwich: 1 piece pita bread stuffed with 6
        tablespoons hummus, 1 cup alfalfa sprouts, and several
        slices roasted red pepper
    1 cup fresh blueberries (or other seasonal fruit)

MIDAFTERNOON SNACK
    1 cup soy milk blended with 1 frozen banana

DINNER
    4 ounces broiled beef tenderloin
    1 medium baked potato
    1 serving tossed salad
    2 tablespoons low-fat Italian dressing

Daily Nutrition Profile: *1371 calories, 19 percent protein, 59 percent carbohydrate, 22 percent fat, 267 milligrams vitamin C, and 22 grams dietary fiber.*

DAY 4

BREAKFAST
    1 cup cooked oat bran
    1 cup fresh blackberries (or other seasonal fruit)
    1 cup skim milk
    1 cup herbal tea

MIDMORNING SNACK
    1 cup vegetable juice

LUNCH
    1 cup low-fat vegetarian chili
    1 serving tossed salad
    2 tablespoons low-fat French dressing

MIDAFTERNOON SNACK
    1 cup cubed watermelon (or other seasonal fruit)

DINNER
    5 ounces roasted turkey breast
    1 cup cooked asparagus spears
    ½ cup sliced boiled beets

Daily Nutrition Profile: *916 calories, 34 percent protein, 54 percent carbohydrate, 11 percent fat, 237 milligrams vitamin C, and 32 grams dietary fiber.*

DAY 5

BREAKFAST
  3 scrambled egg whites
  1 bran muffin
  1 cup fresh raspberries (or other seasonal fruit)
  1 cup herbal tea

MIDMORNING SNACK
  2 low-sodium rice cakes
  1 ounce fat-free Swiss cheese

LUNCH
  8 tablespoons hummus
  1 sliced fresh cucumber (serve hummus on cucumber
    slices)
  1 raw carrot

MIDAFTERNOON SNACK
  1 cup plain nonfat yogurt
  1 tablespoon low-calorie strawberry preserves

DINNER
  Salade Niçoise: 3 ounces water-packed tuna, 1 cup lettuce,
    1 cup chilled whole green beans, 3 small chilled boiled
    potatoes, 3 black olives, and 2 tablespoons low-fat
    Italian dressing
  1 cup honeydew melon balls

Daily Nutrition Profile: 1129 calories, 26 percent protein, 51 percent carbohydrate, 23 percent fat, 128 milligrams vitamin C, and 20 grams dietary fiber.

DAY 6

BREAKFAST
  1 3-inch oat bran bagel
  2 tablespoons fat-free strawberry cream cheese

3 dried figs
1 cup herbal tea

MIDMORNING SNACK
1 cup carrot juice

LUNCH
3 ounces grilled or broiled chicken breast
1 serving tossed salad
2 tablespoons low-fat Italian dressing
½ cup cooked brown rice

MIDAFTERNOON SNACK
Soy shake: 1 cup soy milk blended with 1 cup frozen
   unsweetened strawberries or other frozen unsweetened
   fruit

DINNER
4 ounces baked cod
½ cup lima beans
½ cup cooked corn

*Daily Nutrition Profile: 1301 calories, 31 percent protein, 53
percent carbohydrate, 15 percent fat, 148 milligrams vitamin C,
and 26 grams dietary fiber.*

DAY 7

BREAKFAST
Southern-style breakfast: 2 scrambled eggs, ½ cup corn
   grits, 1 slice turkey ham
1 cup cranberry juice
1 cup herbal tea

MIDMORNING SNACK
1 medium apple

LUNCH
1 cup cooked eggplant with 8 tablespoons spaghetti sauce, and 2 ounces grated fat-free mozzarella cheese

MIDAFTERNOON SNACK
1 cup plain nonfat yogurt with 1 tablespoon low-calorie strawberry preserves

DINNER
5 ounces roasted chicken breast
1/2 cup cooked yams
1 cup cooked spinach

Daily Nutrition Profile: *1286 calories, 32 percent protein, 47 percent carbohydrate, 21 percent fat, 147 milligrams vitamin C, and 12 grams dietary fiber.*

DAY 8

BREAKFAST
1/2 cup All-Bran cereal
1 cup soy milk
1/2 grapefruit
1 cup herbal tea

MIDMORNING SNACK
1 cup sliced cucumbers dipped in 4 tablespoons cottage cheese

LUNCH
1 Greek-style pita pocket sandwich: 1 piece pita bread, 2 ounces feta cheese, 1 cup alfalfa or broccoli sprouts, 2 tablespoons chopped fresh onion, 2 sliced artichoke hearts, and 2 tablespoons low-fat Italian dressing
1 cup low-fat fruit-flavored yogurt

MIDAFTERNOON SNACK
1 banana

DINNER
>   3 ounces pot roast
>   ½ cup peas and carrots medley
>   ½ cup boiled onions

Daily Nutrition Profile: *1258 calories, 24 percent protein, 53 percent carbohydrate, 23 percent fat, 107 milligrams vitamin C, and 31 grams dietary fiber.*

DAY 9

BREAKFAST
>   Yogurt smoothie: Blend 1 cup low-fat plain yogurt with ½ cup orange juice and 1 cup frozen unsweetened strawberries (or other frozen unsweetened fruit).
>   1 cup herbal tea

MIDMORNING SNACK
>   1 cup vegetable juice

LUNCH
>   1 extra-lean hamburger patty
>   Mediterranean salad: 1 cup cooked bulgur wheat, 4 tablespoons chopped parsley, 2 tablespoons chopped onion, and 1 tablespoon olive oil

MIDAFTERNOON SNACK
>   2 low-sodium rice cakes topped with 2 tablespoons cottage cheese with fruit

DINNER
>   4 ounces baked ocean perch
>   1 cup cauliflower
>   1 cup stewed tomatoes

Daily Nutrition Profile: *1144 calories, 27 percent protein, 45 percent carbohydrate, 28 percent fat, 270 milligrams vitamin C, and 20 grams dietary fiber.*

DAY 10

BREAKFAST
  2 shredded wheat biscuits
  1 cup skim milk
  1 sliced banana
  1 cup herbal tea

MIDMORNING SNACK
  1 granola bar

LUNCH
  Low-fat deli sandwich: 2 slices turkey ham, 1 ounce low-fat/low-sodium Swiss cheese, tomato slices, 1 lettuce leaf, 1 tablespoon brown mustard, 2 slices mixed-grain bread

MIDAFTERNOON SNACK
  1 cup carrot juice

DINNER
  1 cup low-fat vegetarian chili
  1 serving tossed salad
  2 tablespoons low-fat French dressing

Daily Nutrition Profile: 1204 calories, 21 percent protein, 63 percent carbohydrate, 16 percent fat, 110 milligrams vitamin C, and 40 grams dietary fiber.

DAY 11

BREAKFAST
  Tropical protein shake: Blend together 1 scoop protein powder, 1 cup skim milk, 1 sliced frozen banana, $\frac{1}{2}$ cup pineapple chunks (juice pack).
  1 cup herbal tea

MIDMORNING SNACK
  2 flavored rice cakes

LUNCH

Chicken Caesar salad: 1 cup shredded romaine lettuce, 3 ounces cubed grilled chicken breast, 2 tablespoons chopped onion, 1 chopped green pepper, 1 tablespoon low-fat Caesar dressing, and 2 tablespoons croutons

MIDAFTERNOON SNACK

1 cup cranberry juice

DINNER

3-ounce extra-lean hamburger patty

1 cup yellow beans

1 cup Brussels sprouts

Daily Nutrition Profile: 1235 calories, 22 percent protein, 48 percent carbohydrate, 31 percent fat, 280 milligrams vitamin C, and 13 grams dietary fiber.

DAY 12

BREAKFAST

1 cup cooked oatmeal

1 cup soy milk

1 fresh orange

1 cup herbal tea

MIDMORNING SNACK

4 Triscuit crackers topped with 2 ounces tofu

LUNCH

European bean salad: 1 cup cooked garbanzo beans, 3 tablespoons chopped onion, 1/2 cup roasted red peppers, and 2 tablespoons low-fat Italian dressing—served on a bed of 3 lettuce leaves.

MIDAFTERNOON SNACK

1/2 cup applesauce

DINNER
   4 ounces grilled salmon
   ¹/₂ cup brown rice
   ¹/₂ cup cooked mushrooms

Daily Nutrition Profile: 1107 calories, 24 percent protein, 52 percent carbohydrate, 24 percent fat, 142 milligrams vitamin C, and 28 grams dietary fiber.

DAY 13

BREAKFAST
   3 scrambled egg whites
   1 cup puffed rice cereal
   1 cup skim milk
   1 cup fresh blueberries (or other seasonal fruit)
   1 cup herbal tea

MIDMORNING SNACK
   1 granola bar
   1 cup melon balls

LUNCH
   Shrimp salad: 3 ounces cooked shrimp, 3 tablespoons
      chopped onion, 4 lettuce leaves, and 1 tablespoon low-
      fat mayonnaise
   2 low-sodium rice cakes

MIDAFTERNOON SNACK
   1 cup carrot juice

DINNER
   4 ounces baked turkey breast
   ¹/₂ cup cooked winter squash
   ¹/₂ cup peas

Daily Nutrition Profile: 970 calories, 35 percent protein, 55 percent carbohydrate, 10 percent fat, 131 milligrams vitamin C, and 20 grams dietary fiber.

DAY 14

BREAKFAST
1 3.5-inch cinnamon-raisin bagel
1 cup plain nonfat yogurt sweetened with 1 tablespoon
 low-calorie strawberry preserves
1 cup calcium-fortified orange juice
1 cup herbal tea

MIDMORNING SNACK
1 raw carrot
2 ounces fat-free cheddar cheese

LUNCH
Fast-food lunch: chicken salad with 2 tablespoons low-fat
 French dressing

MIDAFTERNOON SNACK
1 cup fresh raspberries (or other seasonal fruit) topped
 with 2 tablespoons light nondairy whipped topping

DINNER
1 cup low-fat vegetarian chili
1 serving tossed green salad
2 tablespoons low-fat Italian dressing

Daily Nutrition Profile: *1129 calories, 29 percent protein, 59
percent carbohydrate, 12 percent fat, 237 milligrams vitamin C,
and 33 grams dietary fiber.*

DAY 15

BREAKFAST
Quick smoothie: Blend together 1 packet Carnation Instant
 Breakfast (vanilla flavored), 1 cup skim milk, and 1 cup
 frozen unsweetened strawberries.
1 cup herbal tea

MIDMORNING SNACK
  1 granola bar

LUNCH
  Tuna salad: 3 ounces water-packed tuna, 1 sliced tomato,
    6 lettuce leaves, and 1 tablespoon low-fat mayonnaise.
  1 cup orange sections

MIDAFTERNOON SNACK
  1 cup vegetable juice

DINNER
  4-ounce grilled steak
  1 medium baked potato topped with 1 tablespoon sour
    cream
  1 cup boiled cabbage

*Daily Nutrition Profile: 1050 calories, 34 percent protein, 53
percent carbohydrate, 13 percent fat, 268 milligrams vitamin C,
and 21 grams dietary fiber.*

DAY 16

BREAKFAST
  1 cup plain nonfat yogurt mixed with 1 ounce granola
  1 cup water-packed fruit salad
  1 cup herbal tea

MIDMORNING SNACK
  1 cup sliced cucumbers dipped in 4 tablespoons low-fat
    cottage cheese

LUNCH
  Egg salad pita sandwich: Mix together 2 hard-boiled eggs,
    1 tablespoon low-fat mayonnaise, and 1 teaspoon yellow
    mustard, and spread inside 1 piece pita bread (halved).
    Insert 1 cup alfalfa or broccoli sprouts inside sandwich.
  1 cup raw broccoli pieces

MIDAFTERNOON SNACK
    Fruit smoothie: Blend together 1 cup frozen peaches with
      1 cup skim milk.

DINNER
    4 ounces broiled haddock
    1 cup cooked asparagus

Daily Nutrition Profile: *995 calories, 34 percent protein, 47 percent carbohydrate, 20 percent fat, 153 milligrams vitamin C, and 14 grams dietary fiber.*

DAY 17

BREAKFAST
    2 ounces Cracklin' Oat Bran cereal
    1 cup soy milk
    1 cup fresh blueberries (or other seasonal fruit)
    1 cup herbal tea

MIDMORNING SNACK
    1 energy bar
    1 cup plain nonfat yogurt

LUNCH
    Fast-food lunch: Chicken salad with 2 tablespoons low-fat
      French dressing

MIDAFTERNOON SNACK
    1 medium apple

DINNER
    1 cup low-fat lentil soup
    Caesar salad: 2 cups romaine lettuce, 6 tablespoons grated
      carrot, 1/2 cucumber (sliced), and 1 tablespoon low-fat
      Caesar dressing

Daily Nutrition Profile: 1292 calories, 23 percent protein, 53 percent carbohydrate, 24 percent fat, 111 milligrams vitamin C, and 37 grams dietary fiber.

DAY 18

BREAKFAST
- $^1/_2$ cup cream of wheat cereal
- 1 cup skim milk
- 1 cup melon balls (or other seasonal fruit)
- 1 cup herbal tea

MIDMORNING SNACK
- 1 medium orange

LUNCH
- Deli sandwich: 2 slices reduced-fat ham, 1 ounce low-fat/low sodium Swiss cheese, lettuce leaves, 1 tablespoon brown mustard, and 2 slices light rye bread
- 1 cup raw chopped cauliflower

MIDAFTERNOON SNACK
- 1 serving nutritional beverage such as Boost or Ensure

DINNER
- 4 ounces grilled chicken breast
- 1 cup sliced beets
- 1 serving tossed salad
- 2 tablespoons low-calorie blue cheese dressing

Daily Nutrition Profile: 1203 calories, 26 percent protein, 52 percent carbohydrate, 22 percent fat, 220 milligrams vitamin C, and 19 grams dietary fiber.

DAY 19

BREAKFAST
1 cup cooked oat bran topped with 2 tablespoons wheat germ
1 cup skim milk
1 banana
1 cup herbal tea

MIDMORNING SNACK
3 tablespoons sunflower seeds
1 small packet raisins

LUNCH
Spinach salad: 2 cups fresh spinach, 3 tablespoons chopped onion, 1/2 cup raw sliced mushrooms, 2 ounces tofu, 1/2 cup chilled green beans, and 2 tablespoons low-fat Italian dressing

MIDAFTERNOON SNACK
1 energy bar
1 cup skim milk

DINNER
4 ounces roasted turkey breast
1/2 cup cooked carrots

Daily Nutrition Profile: 1255 calories, 29 percent protein, 49 percent carbohydrate, 23 percent fat, 65 milligrams vitamin C, and 20 grams dietary fiber.

DAY 20

BREAKFAST
Low-fat French toast: Mix together 1 egg, 1 banana, and 1 cup skim milk. Soak two slices cracked-wheat bread in batter and cook until brown on both sides in a skillet coated with nonstick vegetable spray.

2 tablespoons light or no-sugar pancake syrup
1 cup herbal tea

MIDMORNING SNACK
2 rice cakes
2 ounces fat-free cheddar cheese

LUNCH
1 cup low-fat vegetarian chili
1 raw carrot

MIDAFTERNOON SNACK
1 cup fresh raspberries (or other seasonal fruit)

DINNER
4 ounces steamed shrimp
½ cup lima beans
1 corn bread muffin

Daily Nutrition Profile: *1262 calories, 28 percent protein, 61 percent carbohydrate, 11 percent fat, 72 milligrams vitamin C, and 39 grams dietary fiber.*

DAY 21

BREAKFAST
Vegetable omelet: Whisk together 4 egg whites, 1 tablespoon chopped onion, 1 tablespoon chopped green pepper, 2 tablespoons chopped tomatoes, and 1 ounce fat-free cheddar cheese. Cook until firm in an omelet pan or saucepan.
1 slice cracked-wheat bread—toasted
½ grapefruit
1 cup herbal tea

MIDMORNING SNACK
1 cup nonfat or sugar-free fruit-flavored yogurt

LUNCH
   3 ounces grilled chicken breast
   1 serving tossed salad
   2 tablespoons low-fat French dressing

MIDAFTERNOON SNACK
   Fruit smoothie: Blend together 1 cup skim milk with 1 cup
      frozen unsweetened strawberries (or other frozen
      unsweetened fruit).

DINNER
   4 ounces extra-lean hamburger
   1 cup stewed tomatoes
   ½ cup cooked corn

Daily Nutrition Profile: *1265 calories, 33 percent protein, 45
percent carbohydrate, 22 percent fat, 218 milligrams vitamin C,
and 13 grams dietary fiber.*

DAY 22

BREAKFAST
   1 poached egg
   ½ cup All-Bran cereal
   1 cup skim milk
   ½ grapefruit
   1 cup herbal tea

MIDMORNING SNACK
   1 medium apple

LUNCH
   Mexican lunch: 2 corn tortillas filled with 6 tablespoons
      black beans, 2 tablespoons chopped onion, 1 tablespoon
      chopped green pepper, 2 tablespoons chopped tomato,
      and 2 tablespoons salsa
   ½ cup water-packed fruit salad

MIDAFTERNOON SNACK
    1 cup plain nonfat yogurt
    1 tablespoon low-calorie strawberry preserves

DINNER
    4 ounces grilled red snapper
    Caesar salad: 2 cups chopped romaine lettuce, 6
        tablespoons shredded raw carrot, ½ cup chopped
        cucumber, and 1 tablespoon low-fat Caesar dressing

*Daily Nutrition Profile: 1174 calories, 26 percent protein, 60
percent carbohydrates, 15 percent fat, 218 milligrams vitamin
C, and 37 grams dietary fiber.*

DAY 23

BREAKFAST
    1 granola bar
    1 cup soy milk
    1 banana
    1 cup herbal tea

MIDMORNING SNACK
    2 ounces fat-free cheddar cheese

LUNCH
    3 ounces water-packed tuna with 2 cups lettuce, 1 sliced
        tomato, and 2 tablespoons low-fat French dressing
    3 dried figs

MIDAFTERNOON SNACK
    1 cup sugar-free nonfat fruit-flavored yogurt

DINNER
    1 cup low-fat vegetarian lentil chili
    1 cup cooked broccoli
    ½ cup water-packed fruit salad

Daily Nutrition Profile: *1071 calories, 27 percent protein, 60 percent carbohydrate, 13 percent fat, 191 milligrams vitamin C, and 19 grams dietary fiber.*

DAY 24

BREAKFAST
  1 ounce granola mixed in 1 cup plain nonfat yogurt
  1 cup cranberry juice
  1 cup herbal tea

MIDMORNING SNACK
  4 dried apricots

LUNCH
  Gourmet sandwich: 2 ounces goat cheese, lettuce, and 2
    slices enriched French bread. Drizzle with 1 tablespoon
    low-fat French or Italian dressing.
  1 cup fresh strawberries (or other seasonal fruit)

MIDAFTERNOON SNACK
  1 energy bar

DINNER
  Veggie plate: 1 cup cooked mixed vegetables, 1 cup
    cooked corn, and ½ cup brown rice

Daily Nutrition Profile: *1349 calories, 14 percent protein, 68 percent carbohydrate, 18 percent fat, 204 milligrams vitamin C, and 25 grams dietary fiber.*

DAY 25

BREAKFAST
  ½ cup Bran Buds cereal
  1 cup skim milk
  1 cup cantaloupe (or other seasonal fresh fruit)
  1 cup herbal tea

MIDMORNING SNACK
1 apple

LUNCH
3 ounces grilled chicken breast
1 cup cooked broccoli
1 medium baked potato

MIDAFTERNOON SNACK
1 cup plain nonfat yogurt
1 tablespoon low-calorie strawberry preserves

DINNER
4 ounces grilled salmon
Caesar salad: 2 cups shredded romaine lettuce, 1 chopped
tomato, 4 tablespoons chopped onion, 1 grated carrot,
and 1 tablespoon low-fat Caesar dressing.

Daily Nutrition Profile: *1236 calories, 28 percent protein, 56 percent carbohydrate, 17 percent fat, 296 milligrams vitamin C, and 33 grams dietary fiber.*

DAY 26

BREAKFAST
1 cup cooked oatmeal
1 cup skim milk
1 cup fresh strawberries (or other seasonal fruit)
1 cup herbal tea

MIDMORNING SNACK
1 banana

LUNCH
1 cup black bean soup
1 serving tossed salad
1 tablespoon low-fat blue cheese dressing

MIDAFTERNOON SNACK
   1 cup sugar-free nonfat fruit-flavored yogurt

DINNER
   4 ounces grilled chicken breast
   1 cup cooked broccoli
   1 medium sweet potato

Daily Nutrition Profile: *1131 calories, 21 percent protein, 63 percent carbohydrate, 16 percent fat, 264 milligrams vitamin C, and 17 grams dietary fiber.*

DAY 27

BREAKFAST
   Fruit smoothie: Blend together 1 cup nutritional beverage
      such as Boost or Ensure with 1 cup frozen blueberries.
   1 cup herbal tea

MIDMORNING SNACK
   1 oat bran muffin
   1 cup skim milk

LUNCH
   Low-fat chef salad: 1 ounce fat-free cheddar cheese, 2
      slices low-fat ham, 1 chopped tomato, 1 cup raw
      broccoli, 2 cups lettuce, and 2 tablespoons low-fat
      French dressing

MIDAFTERNOON SNACK
   1 medium apple

DINNER
   4 ounces roasted turkey breast
   ½ cup mashed potatoes
   1 cup peas and onions

Daily Nutrition Profile: *1124 calories, 29 percent protein, 62 percent carbohydrate, 9 percent fat, 148 milligrams vitamin C, and 24 grams dietary fiber.*

DAY 28

BREAKFAST
Homemade fast-food breakfast muffin: 2 scrambled egg whites and 1 slice low-fat ham on 1 English muffin
1 cup cranberry juice
1 cup herbal tea

MIDMORNING SNACK
1 serving nutritional beverage such as Boost or Ensure

LUNCH
Mediterranean salad: ½ cup garbanzo beans, 1 ounce feta cheese, 3 tablespoons chopped onion, ½ cup roasted sweet red peppers, 2 cups lettuce, and 2 tablespoons low-fat Italian dressing

MIDAFTERNOON SNACK
1 cup fresh raspberries topped with 2 tablespoons light nondairy whipped topping

DINNER
4 ounces broiled haddock
1 cup cooked carrots
1 cup cooked kale

Daily Nutrition Profile: *1190 calories, 24 percent protein, 61 percent carbohydrate, 15 percent fat, 269 milligrams vitamin C, and 26 grams dietary fiber.*

DAY 29

BREAKFAST
$^1\!/_2$ cup All-Bran
1 cup soy milk
1 cup fresh blackberries (or other seasonal fruit)
1 cup herbal tea

MIDMORNING SNACK
1 fruit/oat bran bar

LUNCH
Tuna pita pocket sandwich: 3 ounces water-packed tuna
  mixed with 1 tablespoon low-fat mayonnaise and 1
  tablespoon sweet relish, and spread inside 1 piece pita
  bread. Stuff sandwich with 1 cup alfalfa or broccoli
  sprouts.
1 medium peach

MIDAFTERNOON SNACK
1 serving energy drink such as Boost or Ensure

DINNER
1 slice roast beef (about 3 ounces)
$^1\!/_2$ cup mashed winter squash
1 cup asparagus

Daily Nutrition Profile: *1239 calories, 28 percent protein, 55
percent carbohydrate, 17 percent fat, 126 milligrams vitamin C,
and 36 grams dietary fiber.*

DAY 30

BREAKFAST
3 scrambled egg whites
1 oat bran muffin
$^1\!/_2$ cup pineapple
1 cup herbal tea

MIDMORNING SNACK
   1 energy bar

LUNCH
   1 cup vegetarian vegetable soup
   1 serving tossed salad
   1 tablespoon low-calorie French dressing
   2 fresh apricots

MIDAFTERNOON SNACK
   1 cup sugar-free nonfat fruit-flavored yogurt

DINNER
   4 ounces grilled chicken breast
   1 medium baked potato with 1 tablespoon fat-free sour
      cream
   1 cup cooked broccoli

Daily Nutrition Profile: *1231 calories, 27 percent protein, 57 percent carbohydrate, 17 percent fat, 146 milligrams vitamin C, and 23 grams dietary fiber.*

PART IV

Anticellulite Exercise

CHAPTER 9

Downsize Your Thighs

•

If you are not already exercising, it's time to start in order to reduce unsightly cellulite. If you are exercising, you probably need to revamp your workout to specifically attack cellulite-affected tissue. Shaping a cellulite-resistant figure requires a three-prong exercise strategy:

- strength training
- stretching
- aerobic exercise

But don't worry! This doesn't mean you must spend more time exercising! Each of these forms of exercise can be incorporated into a *single* workout session. Further, the minimum amount of time you should devote to anticellulite exercising is a mere three hours a week.

In this chapter, we'll examine the importance of strength training to a cellulite-resistant body and how it *spot-tones* your figure and *spot-reduces* cellulite-prone areas, specifically thighs, hips, and buttocks. Strength training is a type of weight-bearing activity in which your muscles are challenged to work harder each time they're exercised. Examples of strength training include lifting weights, working out on weight-training machines, and exercising with special rubber cords or bands.

How Strength Training Reduces and Controls Cellulite

Strength Training Helps You Spot-Reduce

Spot reduction refers to the ability of exercise to scale down selected areas of the body. Quite probably, you've heard that spot reduction isn't possible—that when you exercise, you use energy by metabolizing fat from all over the body, not just from specific areas being worked. That's a true statement. However, blood circulation to fatty, cellulite-prone areas of the body is sluggish. Consequently, fat is more difficult to metabolize in those spots. Strength training to the rescue! By targeting specific body parts, strength training increases circulation in fat storage areas and thus may help to pry loose that stubborn fat.

As a point of fact, spot reduction actually does work—science says so. In one study, when thirty-two subjects strength-trained one arm each day but not the other, they reduced the subcutaneous fat in their exercised arms only. The researchers noted that "fat disappears in areas where muscles are active." So if fat can vanish in exercised regions of the arm, it can probably do so elsewhere on the body—including thighs, hips, and buttocks—with the appropriate type of exercise. That exercise is strength training.

Strength Training Helps You Spot-Tone

By selecting specific exercises, you can spot-tone your thighs, hips, buttocks, and other parts—and remodel your entire figure in the process. Strength training tones your muscles by causing individual muscle fibers to enlarge. This gives your figure the healthy look of firmness, otherwise known as muscle tone. Muscle tone basically means that your muscles are a little larger and more defined.

Understandably, you might be a little reluctant at first to exercise with weights. You're afraid of building bulky muscles.

That's a fear I must dispel. Women simply can't become muscle-bound the way men can. Compared to men, we have about ten times less testosterone, a hormone that causes a male to mature physically and sexually, plus build muscle. Because we have so little of this hormone, we can no more build big muscles than we can grow a beard.

Believe me, it's desirable to build muscle. Developed, toned muscle is what gives your figure noticeable shape and definition. You look leaner, fitter, and more youthful when your muscles are strength-trained.

To spot-tone, you simply target the muscles of those areas in your workout and challenge them accordingly. That way, out-of-shape muscle groups like hips and thighs get extra attention, and soft spots firm up.

Strength Training Burns Fat

Strength training not only gives you a curvier figure, it also helps you get rid of unwanted fat—in three significant ways. First, strength training revs up your metabolism by producing firm, strong muscles that are metabolically active. This means they can burn body fat more efficiently than fat tissue or untoned muscle, even at rest. In addition, the more muscle you have, the faster your metabolic rate, the speed at which chemical reactions like calorie-burning and respiration take place. If you don't have much muscle, your metabolism runs in low gear. Fewer calories are burned, and fat pounds can pile on.

Second, strength training can literally *force fat out of storage depots*. Case in point: A group of women in their seventies started a weight-training program in which they worked their leg muscles only. For purposes of comparison, a control group performed aerobic-type exercise. Prior to the study, the researchers measured the subjects' body composition—lean mass and body fat—in their legs using high-tech computed tomography (also known as a CT scan).

The weight-trained women lost more intramuscular fat (fat that's inside the muscle—like marbling on meat) than the endurance group did. In fact, the researchers noted that fat loss on the endurance-trained women was "negligible." So it appears that you can actually squeeze the fat out with strength training!

Third, strength training turns your muscle fibers into fat-burning units. High-repetition strength training (15 or more repetitions) in particular actually increases the ability of certain types of muscle fibers to burn more fat. Scientists have seen actual proof of this under the microscope by comparing women's muscle tissue before and after a period of high-repetition weight training. In short, strength training turns muscle cells into little burners that incinerate fat.

The message in all this is clear: Strength training is most definitely a fat-burning mode of exercise!

Strength Training Improves Blood and Lymph Circulation

The strength-training exercises you'll perform in the Anticellulite Workout in chapter 12 primarily involve the legs. These exercises force the leg muscles to contract—an action that pushes venous blood and lymph fluid back toward the heart, improving overall circulation.

The same contractive action helps prevent varicose veins—those puffy, twisted blood vessels in the legs that plague many women due to heredity, pregnancy, obesity, and other factors. Strength training, especially when it emphasizes leg work, strengthens leg muscles and turns them into a kind of internal support hose, constantly massaging and protecting the walls of veins.

Strength Training Postpones the Effects of Aging, Including the Development of Cellulite

The loss of muscle tone and strength is a gradual process that begins in your late twenties—unless you undertake a regular exercise program that includes strength training. Strength training is the only exercise known to regenerate vital body tis-

sue (muscle), regardless of age. In one recent study, twenty
people ages fifty-one to eighty-one participated in a twelve-
week strength-training program to see if they could build lean
muscle mass and strength. On average, the women upped their
strength by more than 72 percent; the men by more than 66
percent. These results indicate they were toning and building
precious muscle tissue.

Strength Training Makes You Feel Better About Yourself

The way you think and feel about your appearance is your body
image. If you're like most people, your body image is constantly under attack—mainly by you. Somehow, you're never
quite content with your looks, your size, or your shape. If you
have cellulite, you have probably already given your body low
marks.

By improving your appearance, strength training frees you
from these emotionally harmful dissatisfactions. You'll develop
a renewed appreciation for yourself, for how you look and feel,
and for what you can accomplish.

One intriguing study found that middle-aged and college-
aged women who worked out with weights in a strength-training program significantly improved their self-esteem when
measured against a control group who did not exercise. Researchers Rebecca D. Brown and Joyce M. Harrison noted that
"both the young and mature groups viewed their physical bodies more positively and that their perceptions about themselves
were more positive."

As your outer image begins to improve, so will your inner
image. You'll like the new model, inside and out.

THE BOTTOM LINE

Once you start strength training, your body composition
shifts to firm and away from fat. Muscles that have been toned
through strength training seem to hold any residual body fat in

place better so that it "jiggles" less. Toned muscles also iron out cellulite, thus improving overall skin tone.

The Exercises

The following exercises concentrate on your lower body, mainly the thighs, hips, and buttocks. They are designed to spot-reduce and spot-tone your muscles, plus cellulite-proof your lower body. If you perform these exercises as part of a regular workout program, you'll improve the appearance of your skin and postpone further cellulite development indefinitely.

The Anticellulite Workout in chapter 12 provides directions on the number of repetitions and sets you should perform for each exercise.

BARBELL SQUAT

The barbell squat develops the muscles of your entire lower body, including those of the thighs, hamstrings (the rear of your thighs), hips, buttocks, and calves. The exercise requires the

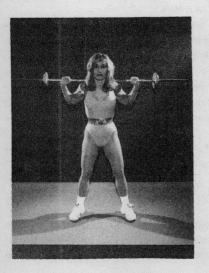

**Barbell Squat
—*Position #1***

Barbell Squat
—*Position #2*

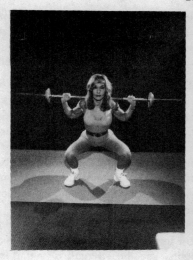

use of a barbell, which is a long, straight metal rod on which iron or vinyl sand-filled plates are attached by collars. These keep the plates from sliding across the bar.

To get the feel of this exercise, use an unloaded bar at first. As you become stronger and more confident in performing the exercise, add a little weight to the bar—perhaps 10 or 15 pounds.

To begin the exercise, place a barbell behind your lower neck so that it is draped just above your rear shoulders. Take an overhand grip on the bar. Your hands should be placed about shoulder-width apart. Your feet should be about 22 to 24 inches apart, with your toes pointed outward. Keep your head up and your back as straight as possible.

Lower your body slowly, until the tops of your thighs are parallel to the floor. Do not go any lower. Using the strength of your thighs, press back up slowly to the starting position. At the top of the movement, squeeze your buttocks together tightly to activate the muscles.

Your repetitions should be kept fairly high (12 to 15), to

accelerate the fat-burning capacity of your muscles. If you own a set of barbells, this exercise can be performed at home.

DUMBBELL BUTTOCKS BURNER

This exercise is a terrific buttocks tightener. It requires the use of dumbbells, which are short bars with adjustable or fixed weights at each end.

Select dumbbells that weigh five to ten pounds. Place two dumbbells about 12 to 18 inches apart on the floor. Stand with your legs comfortably apart. Slowly bend over but keep your head up. Maintain a slight arch in your back and bend your knees slightly. As you bend, get a good stretch in the back of your legs.

At the bottom of the movement, pick up the dumbbells and begin to slowly return to an erect position. While lifting the weights, use the strength of your hips and thighs, not your back. Throughout this portion of the exercise, squeeze your buttocks together as much as possible until you're fully erect.

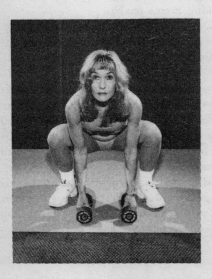

**Dumbbell
Buttocks Burner
—Position #1**

**Dumbbell
Buttocks Burner
—*Position #2***

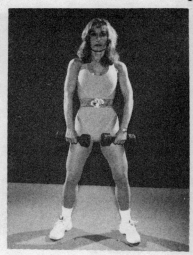

This exercise can also be performed with a barbell, at home if you have a set of weights, or at a gym.

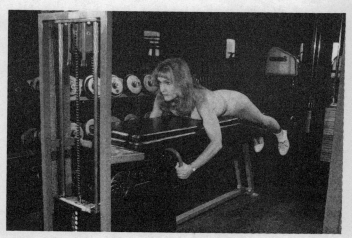

Leg Curl—*Position #1*

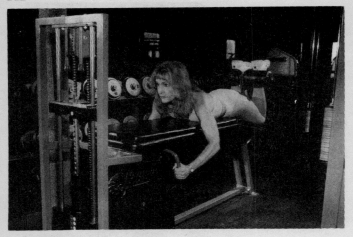

Leg Curl—Position #2

LEG CURLS

Leg curls, which target the hamstrings and buttocks, require a special strength-training machine. It features a padded bench and employs a stack of weights that can be adjusted according to the poundage you want to lift. Adjustments are made by inserting a pin into the stack.

To begin the exercise, select the appropriate poundage by placing the pin in the weight stack. Initially, use a poundage that lets you perform 12 to 15 repetitions without undue strain.

Lie facedown on the machine's padded bench so that your knees and lower legs overhang it slightly. Your kneecaps should not be in contact with the bench. Hook your ankles under the padded roller.

Flex at the knees, bringing your ankles toward your hips in an arc. At the top of the exercise, squeeze your buttocks together. Lower slowly and repeat for the suggested number of repetitions, as specified in the Anticellulite Workout.

**Freehand Squat
—*Position #1***

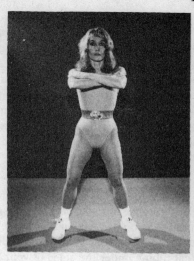

**Freehand Squat
—*Position #2***

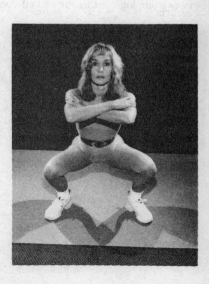

FREEHAND SQUAT

This exercise works the legs and buttocks and requires no special equipment. Stand with your legs a comfortable distance apart and your arms crossed over your chest. Keeping your back straight, squat down until your thighs are just lower than parallel to the floor. Return to the starting position and repeat the exercise as many times as you can. Try to keep constant tension on your thighs and buttocks as you perform this exercise.

CELLULITE BURNER

If this exercise were the only one you ever did, you'd be sure to eradicate cellulite once and for all!

To begin, lie on your back and position an exercise cord or surgical tubing under the soles of your feet. Extend your legs upward so that they are perpendicular to the floor and the soles of your feet are facing the ceiling. Cross the cord in your hands.

Scissor your legs out as far as you can, then bring them to-

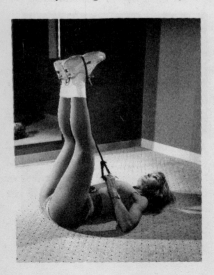

Cellulite Burner —*Position #1*

Cellulite Burner
—*Position #2*

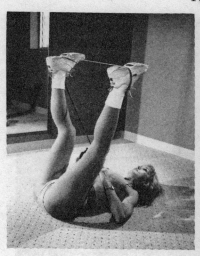

gether again. Repeat this movement as many times as you can. You should feel tension on the backs of your legs, in your inner thighs, and in your buttocks as you perform the exercise.

WALKING DUMBBELL LUNGES

Walking lunges are an excellent shaping and toning exercise for the lower body. To begin, hold a two-, five-, or ten-pound dumbbell in each hand at your sides. While keeping your back straight, step forward on your right leg as far as possible until your right thigh is parallel to the floor. Then bring your left leg forward to meet your right leg.

Next, step forward on your left leg in the same manner and bring your right leg forward to meet your left leg. Continue the exercise by walking forward for about five full minutes, or longer. You can perform this exercise without weights, if you wish.

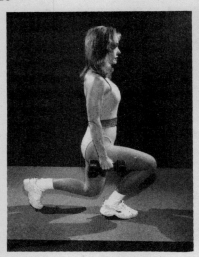

Walking Dumbbell Lunges

LEG EXTENSIONS

This exercise works the frontal portion of your thighs and requires a special apparatus commonly known as a leg extension machine. It is designed with an angled seat, padded rollers, and an adjustable weight stack.

To begin, select an appropriate poundage by placing the pin in the weight stack. Use a poundage with which you can comfortably complete 12 to 15 repetitions during the first set.

Sit in the machine and hook your front ankles under the padded roller. Grasp the handles at the sides of the machine. Extend your lower legs upward in an arc until your legs are straight. Hold your legs in this contracted position for a few seconds.

Slowly lower your legs to the starting position without letting the weight touch the stack. Continue the exercise for the required number of sets and repetitions as outlined in the Anticellulite Workout.

Leg Extension
—*Position #1*

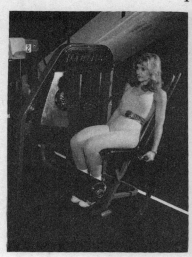

Leg Extension
—*Position #2*

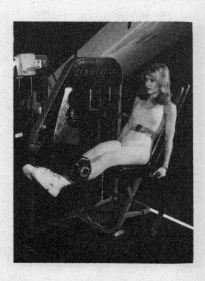

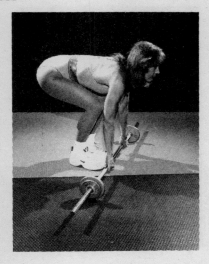

**Straight-Leg Deadlift
—Position #1**

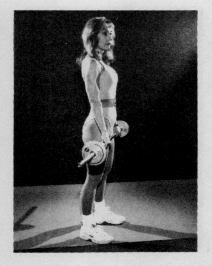

**Straight-Leg Deadlift
—*Position #2***

STRAIGHT-LEG DEADLIFT

This exercise totally isolates the thighs, buttocks, and hamstrings and requires a barbell. Use an unloaded bar, or one that is loaded with no more than 10 pounds if you're just starting to lift weights or 20 pounds if you're already used to lifting weights.

Place the barbell on the floor in front of your feet. To begin the exercise, bend forward and arch your back. This motion isolates your hamstrings. Stretch your hamstrings at the bottom as you pick up the weight. Keeping your legs slightly bent, slowly lift the bar. Pivot at the hip joint and not with your lower back.

At the top of the movement, tighten your buttocks, drive your hips forward, and lock your knees. Then slowly return to the starting position. Repeat the exercise for the required number of sets and repetitions as outlined in the Anticellulite Workout.

Side Lunges

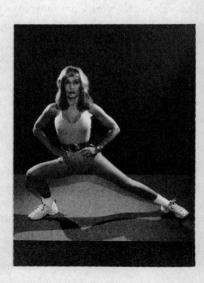

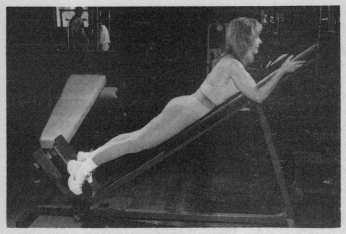

Incline Back Kick—Position #1

SIDE LUNGES

The side lunge works the muscles of the inner thigh, with secondary stress on the frontal thighs. No strength-training equipment is required.

Stand with both feet together. Step sideways into the lunge about two to 2.5 feet, while keeping your other, outstretched leg as straight as you can. Return to the start position and repeat with the other leg. Lunge on each leg for 12 to 15 repetitions.

INCLINE BACK KICK

This exercise firms up the rear of the buttocks and the tops of the hamstrings, an area that tends to sag yet benefits from extra exercise attention. The exercise requires a full-length slant board, which can be found in most gyms and health spas.

Lie face forward on the slant board, and hold on to the edges of the board for support. With your right knee slightly bent,

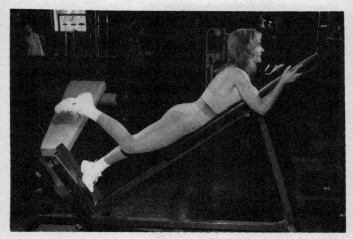

Incline Back Kick—Position #2

raise your right leg up behind you as far as you can. Squeeze your buttocks as tightly as you can. Try to perform as many rep-

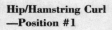

**Hip/Hamstring Curl
—Position #1**

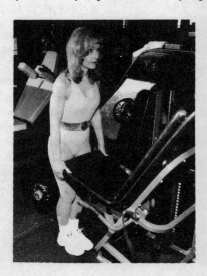

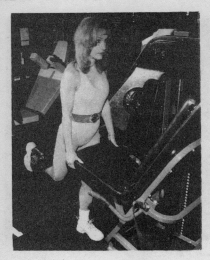

**Hip/Hamstring Curl
—Position #1**

etitions as you can, preferably at the outset and then work up to 25. Repeat the exercise with the left leg.

HIP/HAMSTRING CURL

The point at which the rear of the upper legs meets the lower buttocks is one of the most difficult body spots to develop and tone. This exercise does the trick.

You'll need a leg extension machine to perform it. Stand, facing the seat of the machine, and position your body between the seat and the padded foot roller. One leg at a time will be exercised. Place the lower back part of the exercising leg under the foot roller. Grasp the sides of the seat and lean forward slightly. Curl your leg up toward your buttocks. You should feel a deep, muscle-stimulating burn in your buttocks and hamstrings. Complete the required number of repetitions, then work the other leg in the same manner.

Guidelines for Anticellulite Strength Training

If you're new to strength training, start slowly. For best results, the American College of Sports Medicine recommends strength training two to three times a week.

Initially, you may want to work with a qualified trainer, who can teach you the exercises, help you with proper exercise form, and motivate you to continue your exercise program.

To develop body-firming muscle, you must challenge your muscles to work harder each time you exercise. That means progressively upping your poundages or doing more repetitions from workout to workout. Try to increase poundages by two to ten pounds each time you work out, or add a few extra repetitions to each exercise set.

Before you begin any exercise program, consult your physician and have a complete medical checkup.

Here are some additional pointers:

- When you first try an exercise, use a light weight, one that you can comfortably lift for 12 to 15 repetitions. The last two to three repetitions should feel harder and require extra effort.
- On the lifting and lowering portion of an exercise, control the weight without letting momentum take over.
- Perform two to three sets of each exercise. A set is a series of repetitions.
- Each time you exercise, work your way up. Strive to lift more weight than before, or perform more repetitions. Progression builds strength and develops lean muscle.
- Breathe naturally as you exercise. Never hold your breath.
- Work out two to three times a week on nonconsecutive days. Your muscles need to rest approximately forty-eight hours before being exercised again.

CHAPTER 10

Conditioning Your Connective Tissue

An often overlooked component of exercise is stretching—a slow, sustained elongation of muscle and connective tissue. Done correctly, it can enhance the tone and shape of muscles, which in turn helps smooth out cellulite-ridden skin. Primarily, stretching promotes flexibility, the ability to move joints and muscles easily through their full range of motion.

There are several methods of stretching, and they generally fall into two broad categories: static stretching and dynamic stretching. Dynamic stretching involves bouncing movements that replicate moves employed in certain sports. Gymnasts and skaters are among the athletes who regularly perform dynamic stretching exercises in their training. A variation of dynamic stretching called active stretching or rhythmic limbering is often used in aerobic dance classes as part of the warm-up.

Static stretching is the more familiar of the two. It involves holding a muscle in a stretched position for several seconds and is less stressful on the body than dynamic stretching.

The primary type of stretching to be concerned with for fighting cellulite is fascial stretching, a variation on static stretching developed for bodybuilders by fitness expert and author John Parrillo. Not coincidentally, the physiques of male and female bodybuilders are typically cellulite free!

Understanding this technique starts with some basic anatomy involving the fascia, one of six internal tissues of the body, along with muscles, tendons, bones, joints, and ligaments. It is a thick, fibrous sheet that envelops individual muscles and groups of muscles and, like a divider, separates their layers and groupings. Under the skin, it also separates the subcutaneous fat layer from the deep fat layer. The fascia encloses other structures too, including tendons, joints, blood vessels, nerves, and organs. In fact, there are more than fifty types of fascial tissue throughout the body.

Think of the fascia as a shock absorber for the tissues it surrounds, protecting them from blows of athletics or the stresses of exercise. And what a protector it is: On the molecular level, fascial tissue is stronger than structural steel.

Fascial stretching is designed to improve muscular size, shape, and strength. Stretching the fascia opens up the spaces surrounding a muscle, giving it more room to grow. Inwardly, greater growth leads to firmer, shapelier muscles; outwardly, it produces tighter, smoother skin.

Fascial stretching does not take extra time. In fact, the method involves stretching *between* strength-training sets. Strength training itself stretches the fascia to some degree. But add stretching between sets to your routine, and you stretch the fascia even further.

The benefits of stretching, including fascial stretching, don't end with muscle size and shape. For example:

Stretching Improves Flexibility
Stretching makes your body more flexible, giving your muscles and the joints they connect greater range of motion. With greater range of motion, muscles can exert more power and work harder, leading to greater firmness and strength. What's more, a pliable, flexible physique is less susceptible to injuries because it can better withstand physical stresses.

Stretching Enhances the Health of Connective Tissue

Flexible connective tissue retains its elasticity, an important component of a youthful-looking body. The optimum way to gain and preserve flexibility is through stretching.

Stretching Prevents Muscle Soreness

Stretching may also reduce a condition known as delayed onset muscle soreness (DOMS), the pain and stiffness that occurs in muscles between twenty-four and forty-eight hours after intense or unaccustomed exercise.

Stretching Rids Your Body of Lactic Acid

Stretching loosens tight muscles, which tend to trap lactic acid, a waste product that accumulates in muscle cells during exercise. When lactic acid builds up, muscular fatigue and achiness are the result. Stretching helps release lactic acid from muscle cells into the bloodstream so that it does not interfere with muscular contraction. The loosening effect of stretching also helps you breathe better during workouts. This enhances your oxygen utilization for improved energy levels and greater fat mobilization.

Fascial Stretches for the Lower Body

The following fascial stretches should be performed between strength-training sets and after your strength-training workout. The Anticellulite Workout described in chapter 12 shows you how to incorporate these stretches into a strength-training routine.

THIGH STRETCH

Stand next to a bench or other piece of sturdy gym equipment. Bend your left knee, as illustrated. Holding your left ankle, bring your bent leg behind you. For balance, hold on to the equipment.

Press your left heel to your buttocks while pushing your

Thigh Stretch

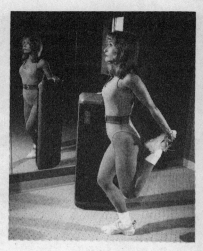

thigh down and back. Hold for ten to 20 seconds, then release. Repeat with the right thigh.

FORWARD HAMSTRING STRETCH

This movement stretches the hamstring muscle at the rear of the thigh. To begin, sit with your legs extended straight out in front of you. Lean forward and clasp the tops of your feet. Make sure your knee joints are locked out tightly.

Pull the tops of your feet toward you. Stretch hard. Hold for a count of ten to 20 seconds before releasing.

HIP STRETCH

Sit on the floor with your legs extended out in front of you. Bend your left leg and cross it over your right leg. Place your elbow on your leg, as illustrated.

Rotate your upper body as far to the left as you can. Turn your shoulders around, pushing your knee over. Balance your-

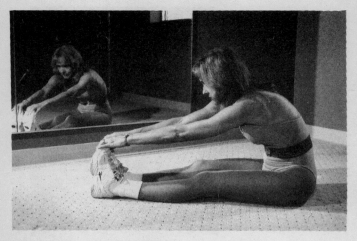

Forward Hamstring Stretch

self with your hands. Hold for ten to 20 seconds, then release. Repeat the stretch with your right leg.

BUTTERFLY

This movement stretches your inner thighs and hips. Sit on the floor with your knees bent and apart, and the bottoms of your feet pressed together, as illustrated.

With your back arched slightly, move your upper body forward while pressing your inner thighs down toward the floor. Hold for a count of ten to 20 seconds.

INNER THIGH/HAMSTRING STRETCHES

There are three variations of this stretch. In the first, sit on the floor with your legs spread as wide apart as possible. Press your upper body toward the floor as you walk forward with your hands as far as you can. Hold for a count of 10 to 20 seconds, then release.

In the second variation, reach over your left leg and grasp

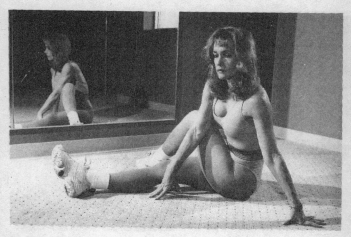

Hip Stretch

your left foot with both hands. Lean toward your foot and stretch hard.

In third variation, grasp both feet with your hands. Lean forward slightly and stretch hard.

Hold these stretches for a count of 10 to 20 seconds, then release.

General Guidelines for Stretching

- Do not bounce your limbs when performing fascial stretching; quick, jerky movements may tighten the muscle rather than relax it.
- Breathe normally. Proper breathing helps your body eliminate lactic acid and other waste products of exercise, plus oxygenates your muscles.
- Do not stretch a cold muscle. Many people mistakenly believe that stretching provides a good warm-up. But if you stretch a cold muscle, you're setting yourself up for injury. Stretch between exercise sets or after your workout

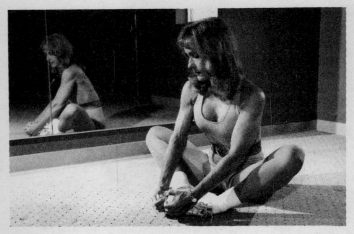

Butterfly

when your muscles are already warm. The best warm-up prior to exercise is a moderate five- to ten-minute walk.

• Stretches such as the ones described above can be performed as a cool-down following your strength-training workout. During this period, your muscles are warm and pliable because blood is still pulsing through them. Postworkout stretching eases muscular tightness brought on by strength-training exercises.

Other Paths to Stretching:
Yoga and Ballet

Yoga and ballet are two forms of stretching-type exercise that promote suppleness, healthy connective tissue, smooth skin, and overall good health. For variety, you may want to try one or the other, or both.

Although practiced for more than five thousand years, yoga is today enjoying a resurgence of popularity, particularly in the United States. It is often used as complementary therapy to

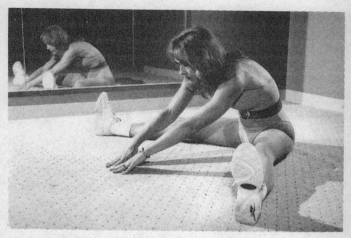

Inner Thigh/Hamstring Stretch—Variation #1

treat patients with respiratory ailments, digestive problems, obesity, and other diseases.

There are many types of yoga, but most fall into the category of hatha yoga. Hatha yoga incorporates an assortment of asanas, or postures. The postures employed are excellent for enhancing blood circulation.

A popular variation of yoga is a type of workout called power yoga. It is more vigorous and emphasizes strength over suppleness. In a power yoga class, you typically perform a sequence of about thirty-two floor exercises that flow from one to the other, much like a dance routine. During each pose, you're instructed to tense, or contract, each muscle as hard as you can. Power yoga doesn't require any special skill or training; just about anyone can do it.

One chief reason yoga and its variations may be good choices for fighting cellulite is that yoga has been shown in research to reduce the thickness of fatty tissue in the thighs, plus pare down the girth of the hips. Other benefits include:

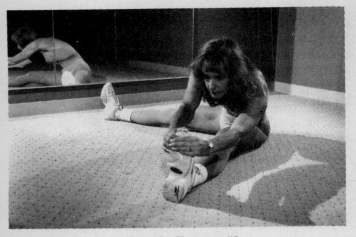

Inner Thigh/Hamstring Stretch—Variation #2

- increased strength
- flexibility
- less stiffness and pain
- a firm and elastic physique
- improved balance
- better posture
- extra energy
- stress relief

Add to the list of cellulite-free bodies those of ballet dancers. Studies of ballet dancers consistently find that they have a smaller percentage of body fat and a greater percentage of muscle than nondancers. If you've ever admired the longer, prettier muscles sported by ballerinas, and want to make your legs sleek rather than sizeable, why not consider taking an adult ballet class?

After years of ballet training as a youngster, I decided in 1999 to resume the discipline, primarily to give my body a different type of physical stress. After only six months of once-a-

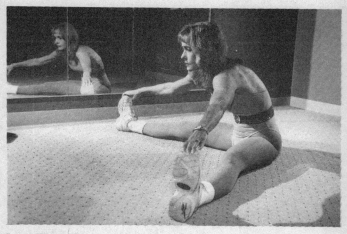

Inner Thigh/Hamstring Stretch—Variation #3

week classes, I noticed that my upper thighs had a more grace-
ful shape than I had been able to attain with strength training.
Now I'm hooked.

Unquestionably, ballet training produces smooth, sculpted
muscles. It also enhances your flexibility, balance, and posture—which all tend to slip with age.

Ballet also:

- increases endurance and strength.
- promotes agility and coordination.
- works large muscle groups such as the thighs and
  buttocks.
- makes the heart beat faster to encourage better circulation.

Some gyms and spas offer ballet-type workouts, which provide the same benefits, while providing more vigorous exercise
moves.

CHAPTER 11

Fat-Burning, Body-Toning Aerobics

Aerobic exercise—the kind that gets your heart pumping—helps strip away body fat to reveal your natural shape and thus is very important for minimizing cellulite. Examples of aerobic exercise include walking, jogging, running, swimming, bicycling, and aerobic dancing. There are enormous anticellulite benefits from this kind of exercise. Consider:

Aerobic Exercise Deflabs Your Figure
Several fat-burning mechanisms are at work when you exercise aerobically. First, your body draws on fat in the form of fatty acids as one of its energy sources. In the first leg of aerobic exercise, your body starts burning mainly carbohydrate for fuel. After about twenty minutes, fat starts to kick in more fuel, especially as you pick up your pace. Further, the more aerobically fit you are, the sooner your body switches over to fat stores and the greater percentage of fat you'll burn for fuel. An aerobically fit body is a fat-burning body.

Second, aerobic exercise also increases fat-burning enzymes in your body. You need those enzymes if you want to become leaner.

Third, aerobic exercise builds the number and density of tiny structures inside cells called mitochondria, where fat and other nutrients are burned. The more mitochondria you have, the more fat your body can burn.

And fourth, aerobic exercise builds your oxygen-processing capacity. Fat is burned only when there's adequate oxygen around.

Aerobic Exercise Stimulates Your Metabolism

A faster, more efficient metabolism accentuates fat-burning. Your metabolic rate (the speed at which your body burns calories) stays elevated during and after aerobic exercise ends. So not only are you burning calories while exercising, you continue to do so later. And the longer your exercise session, the longer your metabolic rate stays up afterward.

Aerobic Exercise Enhances Blood Circulation

Your entire circulatory system changes as a result of aerobic exercise. It makes your capillaries increase in size and number, so that more oxygen and nutrients find their way to the muscles and other tissues (including cellulite-affected tissues) where it's needed. The buildup of muscle capillaries can take place rapidly—within just a few weeks of training.

The Importance of Aerobic Intensity

With aerobic exercise, try to gradually work up to a high-intensity, vigorous pace. Aerobic intensity is typically measured by the rate at which your heart beats while exercising. It's best to exercise at a level that's 65 to 85 percent of your maximum heart rate (MHR). To calculate your MHR, simply subtract your age from 220. Let's say you're forty years old. Your MHR would be 180 (220 − 40). Your "target zone" would be 117 beats per minute (180 × .65) to 153 beats (180 × .85). Exercising in the upper end of your zone will help you burn more

Table 11.1—*Target Heart Rate Zones*

Age	Maximum Heart Rate	85% of Maximum
20	200	170
25	195	166
30	190	162
35	185	157
40	180	153
45	175	149
50	170	145
55	165	140
60	160	136
65	155	132
70	150	128

fat. Table 11.1 will help you find the upper end of your target heart rate zone.

To find your heart rate during exercise, take your pulse at the radial artery in either wrist, or at the carotid artery to the left or right of your windpipe. Place your index and middle finger lightly over the artery. Don't press too hard, particularly on the carotid artery. Too much pressure can actually slow your pulse. Count the beats for ten seconds, then multiply that number by six to get your heart rate for a minute.

An excellent indicator of your aerobic fitness is your heart rate at rest. In a very highly trained aerobic athlete, the heart beats 30 to 40 beats a minute at rest; in normal, healthy people, 70 to 80 beats a minute; and in sedentary and out-of-shape people, 80 to 100 beats a minute. Check your heart rate occasionally when you get up in the morning. If it's low, your heart is beating fewer times but pumping more blood with each beat. That means it's working more efficiently.

The Frequency of Aerobics

You can obtain satisfactory results in terms of fat-burning with two to three aerobic sessions a week. It's generally recognized that the best advances (especially in terms of fat loss) are made by exercising four to five days a week. Of course, frequency depends on your personal schedule. It's not always feasible to fit in five aerobic sessions a week.

The Duration of Aerobics

The longer each aerobic session is, the more fat you'll burn. Remember: After twenty minutes, your body starts relying more on fat for fuel, especially if you're working out in the upper end of your target heart rate zone. So for fat loss, you must try to work out aerobically for longer than twenty minutes. Also, for a conditioning effect on your heart, you need to exercise in your target heart rate zone for at least twenty minutes.

Combine Aerobics with Strength Training

You can multiply your fat-burning power by combining aerobics with strength training. Aerobic exercise burns fat by numerous mechanisms, and strength training burns fat too, but in different ways. So by doing both, you're burning fat not one way but multiple ways! In fact, one study found that people who combined strength-training exercises with aerobics lost 2.5 times more fat!

A convenient, time-saving way to combine the two is to perform aerobic exercise after you strength-train. This sequence has a powerful fat-burning benefit. Here's why: As you strength-train, carbohydrate, in the form of glucose (blood sugar) and glycogen in your muscles, supplies the energy you need for the activity. Following your strength-training routine, your body has less carbohydrate available for energy. If you perform your aerobics *after* your strength-training routine, your body's primary fuel source becomes fat—exactly what you want to burn. Put another way, your body dips into its fat stores earlier because carbohydrate fuel was emptied during the strength-training portion of your workout. In the Anticellulite Workout outlined in the next chapter, I recommend that you follow this sequence for optimal fat-burning.

Best Aerobic Bets to Cast Out Cellulite

Used to be, aerobics was aerobics was aerobics. Not anymore. Today there are special aerobic classes and new machines, which besides their primary heart-pumping action provide fat-burning stimulation to specific parts of the body. However, the very best aerobic program is the one you enjoy—and will stick to.

Here's a look at some of the best aerobic choices available, from the conventional to the high-tech.

Conventional Aerobics

WALKING

Millions of people walk for fitness, pleasure, or both. For aerobic exercise beginners, walking may be the best method of getting in shape. It's easy to do, convenient, and inexpensive. As for aerobic benefits, you can easily reach your target heart rate zone with brisk walking. Walking one mile burns approximately 100 calories. More important, it works the lower body, where cellulite tends to form. If your walking route is hilly, expect your hips and buttocks to get a superintense workout.

When starting a walking program, begin the first week by walking twenty minutes three times a week. For the next few weeks, increase your time to thirty minutes. As you feel more energetic and fit, add an extra session or two to your weekly walking program. Try to work up to five sessions a week, thirty to forty-five minutes each time, especially if you're trying to pare off fat pounds. Remember to walk at a good clip too, in order to keep your heart rate in its target zone.

To burn more calories, try swinging your arms while you walk. Research shows that vigorous arm swinging increases your calorie-burning potential by 50 percent, plus gives your upper body a good workout.

Here are some additional tips:

- Wear sturdy athletic shoes.
- Keep your head level as you walk, and look straight ahead.
- Bend your elbows at about a ninety-degree angle and keep them close to your sides. Swing your arms backward and forward as you walk.
- Let your heel strike the ground first, then roll from the heel to the ball of your foot. Push off with the ball of your foot for more momentum.
- Take long, smooth strides. Walk as briskly as you can.
- Breathe deeply but naturally as you walk.

WEIGHTED WALKING

A variation of walking is to use weights, which are strapped to your ankles, held in your hands, or worn on a belt and attached to your hips and chest. An advantage of weighted walking is that it's a great way to increase your aerobic intensity, particularly if you don't want to jog or run. In one study, researchers demonstrated that the intensity of walking at four miles per hour with ankle and hand weights was comparable to, and, in some cases exceeded, that of running at five miles per hour. Weighted walking burned 120 to 158 calories a mile, whereas running expended 120 to 130 calories a mile.

It's best to begin a weighted walking program without weights, then add them later and start with one-pound weights. Gradually increase weight in one-pound increments until you're carrying about 5 percent of your body weight.

JOGGING AND RUNNING

It's rare to see a runner who has cellulite! Runners are generally lean, with shapely, firm legs. So if you're physically ambitious, you might consider starting a jogging or running program.

The average speed for jogging is about five miles an hour. At higher speeds, you'll find it easier to run. Whether you jog or run, work on covering the same distance in less time. If you decide to run, increase mileage by no more than 10 percent of the previous week's total. Here are some other pointers for jogging and running:

- Wear sturdy, well-cushioned running shoes.
- Run in well-lit areas and let people know your route.
- Run on smooth, well-cushioned tracks rather than on hard pavement.
- Maintain good posture, with your head and chin up.
- Keep your elbows bent in a ninety-degree angle and held close to your side. Let your arms swing backward and forward as you jog or run.
- Take fairly short steps, letting your heel strike first.
- Breathe normally.

BIKING

Outdoor biking is a great fat burner, expending as many as 500 calories an hour. Not only that, it tones up cellulite trouble spots like hips and thighs. But biking requires some skill to maneuver the bicycle safely and competently. If you haven't ridden recently, you'll have to do some practice riding to become familiar with your bike and the proper riding position.

To get the fitness benefits of biking, ride at a speed of ten to fifteen miles per hour on a straight stretch. Begin with about twenty minutes, two or three times the first week. Each week, gradually add to your distance and increase the frequency with which you ride. Don't ride on consecutive days either, since your muscles (particularly your thigh muscles) need time to rest and recover.

There are many safety precautions to heed as an outdoor cyclist. Know the rules of the road, review bicycle safety, wear bright clothing, and always wear a bicycle helmet. Many communities have biking clubs, and these are a good way to master this sport and meet other enthusiasts. Usually, biking shops have information on clubs and how to join them.

Class-Type Aerobics

AEROBIC DANCE CLASSES

For millions of people, aerobic dance classes offer an enjoyable, effective way to get in shape. What's more, you can maximize your fat-burning potential since classes are intense and usually last an hour. Large muscle groups, particularly those of the lower body, are worked fairly hard. Consequently, muscle tone is thus improved and cellulite is minimized.

As with most forms of aerobics, aerobic dancing, done at high intensities, enhances your cardiovascular fitness. Plus, you achieve better coordination, posture, and body carriage, thanks to the often-intricate dance moves taught in classes.

The trend for a long time has been toward nonimpact aerobic dancing. With this form of aerobics, at least one foot touches the floor throughout the aerobic portion of the workout. Dance steps are jumpless, knee lifts replace knee hops, and large upper-body movements with a wide range of motion are used. As a result, nonimpact aerobic dance is thought to be safer, since it eliminates the repetitive pounding on the joints on the dance floor.

Low impact does not necessarily mean low intensity, however. Intensity in low-impact classes is achieved by increasing the amount of work done with the arms, the difficulty of the dance steps, and the cadence of those steps.

Low-impact aerobics does burn fat. One study looked into the effects of this type of workout on fifteen sedentary women, ages thirty-five to sixty-four. The women exercised for ten weeks, without changing or controlling their diets. On average, they lost 2.5 percent body fat over the course of the experimental period.

Whatever class you choose, make sure the instructor is certified to teach aerobics. Also, see that your instructor works closely with you, according to your level of experience, in order to help you progress.

For convenience, you may opt to do aerobic dance at home—with videos. There are hundreds to choose from—so before buying, rent a couple from your local video store or check one out from the library. Make sure the instructor's explanations are easy to understand and that the instructor is a good motivator. The workout should include a warm-up, an aerobic segment that's at least twenty to thirty minutes long, and a cool-down. Also, you can tell a lot about the quality of the exercise program by the quality of the video production.

BENCH STEPPING

For greater aerobic fitness and lower-body-toning action, many classes have added special benches to choreographed routines. As part of the routine, you step up and down on a bench. Benches come in adjustable heights, typically ranging from six to twelve inches tall. The higher the adjustment, the harder and more intense the workout. Often, exercisers use handheld weights to increase the intensity of the effort and burn more calories. Bench stepping is an excellent way to increase blood circulation to the hips, buttocks, and thighs.

In studies, bench stepping has stood up well as an aerobic

exercise, burning more calories than walking. Exercise physiologists agree that it provides sufficient aerobic demand for both cardiovascular fitness and weight loss.

High-Tech Aerobics

CROSSROBICS

Without a doubt, this equipment (from StairMaster) represents a new generation of training—one that combines aerobics and weight training into a single workout.

The machine resembles a recumbent stair climber, but with a weight stack at your right. You can choose various programs, levels of intensity, and duration of exercise. A computerized readout of the program on a panel lets you see the upcoming peaks and valleys.

After the program begins, you push the pedals against resistance. This works your thighs hard! The angled position of your body ensures that your thighs are directly isolated. As you work out, you must keep the weight stack suspended within a specific range. Depending on how you set up your Crossrobics program, the machine will ask you to increase your poundage on the weight stack for greater intensity about midway through the program.

With Crossrobics, you can pursue high-repetition training. This type of training has the potential to increase the number of mitochondria (cellular units that burn fat) in fast-twitch muscle fibers. With more mitochondria, muscle fibers burn more fat. Regular training on Crossrobics could turn your body into a fat- and cellulite-busting machine.

CROSS-COUNTRY SKI SIMULATORS

Few would disagree that cross-country skiing is one of the best aerobic exercises ever. Years ago, innovative manufacturers developed cross-country ski machines, which are available for home use and in health clubs. Though several types are on the market—some computerized—all of the equipment places fitness-building demands on the lower and upper bodies.

With this equipment, you simulate the motion of a cross-country skier, alternating your arms and legs in a forward then backward sliding motion. Some machines provide variability in speed and resistance for a wide range of exercise intensities.

STATIONARY BICYCLES

This high-tech form of aerobics is one of the most popular. It improves your fat-burning capability, increases your lower-body tone, and enhances your aerobic power, provided you exercise in the upper level of your target heart rate zone.

Sometimes boredom is a problem with stationary cycling. Consider pedaling while watching television, or using some of the bike's motivating features—like computerized hill profiles, challenging resistance settings, or touch-screen readouts to monitor your progress—to make the ride more interesting.

When working out on a stationary bicycle, it's important to adjust the seat height correctly. If your seat is too low or too high, your legs won't pedal efficiently, and you could place undue stress on your knee joint. Find the correct seat height by placing one of the pedals in the fully lowered position. Sit on the bike and extend your leg to the pedal, making sure there's a slight bend in your knee. If not, readjust the seat accordingly.

Most stationary cycles have varying levels of difficulty. Initially, start at the lowest. Each week, try to move up to the next level of difficulty. Be sure to take your heart rate before, during, and after your workout. Try to work out in your target heart rate range for at least twenty minutes or longer.

The hottest exercise trend today is Spinning, in which you ride stationary bikes in a class set to music and led by a certified instructor. The instructor takes you through a series of simulated hills, straightaways, and downhills, all made easy or tough by changing the resistance on your bike. Spinning classes are much more intense than riding a stationary bike on your own. Plus, they work the muscles of your hips and thighs extremely hard.

RECUMBENT STATIONARY BICYCLES

With this version of a stationary bike, you're seated so that your legs are parallel to the floor. In this position, the recumbent bike does a better job of isolating the thighs than a conventional stationary bike does. Once you start pedaling, practically all you feel is a leg-pumping burn.

Depending on the product, there's generous support for your hips, pelvis, and lower back, along with an extra-wide seat. Electronic models incorporate various levels of difficulty and intensity, giving you opportunities to do more each time you exercise.

SLIDE EXERCISING

This activity incorporates a flexible board slightly over six feet long, with a special laminated surface. Simulating the motion of speed skating or roller skating, you actually slide on the device from side to side for a great lower-body workout. It helps to wear the "sliders" that fit over your athletic footwear and provide the right amount of friction for the exercise.

In university tests, the caloric cost of using this apparatus was found to be 20 percent greater than performing a standard aerobics workout, and 16 percent higher than riding a stationary bicycle. A ten-minute workout on the slide expends 74 calories. To use up the same amount of calories while doing aerobics, you would have to exercise 12.7 minutes longer; while riding a stationary bike, 12.1 minutes longer. In other words, you can burn more calories in less time compared to other forms of aerobics.

This type of workout has been used for years by professional skaters to condition their upper and lower bodies. Ideal for home aerobics use, this apparatus is available in sporting goods stores nationwide and at a reasonable cost. Some aerobic dance classes incorporate slide exercising into their routines.

STAIR-CLIMBING MACHINES

Like many mechanized aerobic machines, stair climbers provide instant feedback on calories burned, heart rate, and other variables. You can set the level of difficulty too. These machines work the large muscles of the lower body, adding to the intensity of the effort. Leg strength and muscle tone can increase too.

Research shows that these devices do an excellent job of boosting aerobic power. In one study, fifteen women between the ages of twenty-five and forty-eight worked out on a stair climber at moderately high intensities for thirty minutes three times a week for twelve weeks. After the study, their aerobic power had increased by 36 percent, an improvement that matches increases reported for walking, running, and cycling.

Experts advise that workouts on these machines should be performed in the lower end of your target heart rate zone. That's a little less than advised for other aerobic workouts, but these machines can overstress heart, lungs, and muscles if you push it too much. Plus, your muscles can fatigue too early, since there's resistance supplied by the machine. If you fizzle out too early, you'll miss out on the fat-burning benefits of stair climbing.

TREADMILLS

Among the best aerobic cellulite reducers is the treadmill. According to one impressive scientific study, people who ran on treadmills lost more fat from their hips, rear thighs, and buttocks (all cellulite-prone spots) than anywhere else on their bodies.

Treadmills provide a great way for you to walk, jog, or run indoors, at home or in a gym. You can adjust the speed of the treadmill according to your level of fitness, and increase the speed gradually as you become more conditioned. The grade or slope of the treadmill can also be adjusted to make the exercise feel harder, like you're jogging or running uphill. Some computerized treadmills let you choose certain programs in which the speed and grade automatically change while you're on the machine. Don't forget to monitor your heart rate.

Aerobic Exercise Guidelines

No matter what type of aerobic activity you choose, it should start with a warm-up and finish with a cool-down. The warm-up is light activity performed for five to ten minutes—walking at a slow pace, pedaling against very light resistance, slow stepping on a stair-climbing machine, and so forth. The warm-up decreases stress on your heart, lowers your blood pressure, increases blood flow, and keeps your joints and muscles limber.

Similarly, a cool-down is five to ten minutes of less vigorous activity—either walking or stretching—to help your heart rate return to normal. It also removes exercise-generated waste products from your muscles and keeps blood from pooling in your legs. If blood is allowed to collect in your legs, blood pressure can drop sharply, possibly causing dizziness. The cool-down keeps blood circulating back toward the heart. Don't ever neglect either the warm-up or cool-down; make them essential parts of your aerobic workout.

Mix It Up for Motivation

One way to stay motivated in your aerobic exercise program is to combine various types of aerobics using a cross-training approach. For example, you might try this routine:

- five minutes of walking around an indoor track (warm-up)
- ten to fifteen minutes on a stair-climbing machine
- ten to fifteen minutes on a rowing machine

- ten to fifteen minutes on a stationary bicycle
- five minutes of walking around an indoor track (cool-down)

There are other combinations you can try too. Whatever aerobic activity you pursue, be sure to keep track of your heart rate, and the duration and frequency of your workouts. That way, you can ensure that you're making steady progress.

CHAPTER 12

The Anticellulite Workout

The Anticellulite Workout described below is designed to trim your legs and buttocks, firm up muscle, and smooth out cellulite. It employs simple, easy-to-perform exercises, which were described in chapters 9 and 10. The easier the exercises, the more likely you are to stick with the workout and enjoy yourself while following it.

The workout employs a variety of equipment, each designed for a specific task. Barbells and dumbbells—known as free weights—are superior for firming up muscle and building strength in the shortest possible time. A barbell is a long, straight metal rod on which iron plates are attached by collars. These keep the plates from sliding across the bar. Dumbbells are simply shorter versions of barbells and are used to isolate and define specific muscles. Barbell and dumbbell exercises can be performed at home, as well as at a gym.

Machines are pieces of weight-training equipment with weight stacks that can be adjusted according to the poundage you want to lift. Adjustments are made by inserting a pin into the stack. Leg curl and leg extension machines are two examples of weight stack machines.

Exercise Performance

With this workout, the way you execute each strength-training repetition makes the difference between results that are pleasing and results that are just mediocre. By performing every repetition correctly, you work your muscle fibers completely and efficiently, resulting in muscular tone, shape, and strength.

A repetition is the path of an exercise from the start of the movement to the midpoint and back again to the start position. Sounds simple enough, but in reality there's a lot that goes into performing repetitions correctly. Here are some pointers:

- **Style.** Always control the motion of the exercise. A mistake many exercisers make is starting the exercise with a rapid, jerky movement. This action gives the weight so much impetus that it practically glides to the midpoint of the rep, using little muscular force to get there. As a result, the muscles encounter limited resistance. Without resistance, muscles aren't properly challenged and may not respond as well.

  The correct way to start the repetition is to gradually apply the sheer force of your muscles to lift the weight. If you can't lift the weight without jerking it, then your poundage is too heavy. Try a lighter weight. Strict style and technique are more important than the amount of weight you lift.

- **Speed.** "Slow" is the watchword here. Both the raising motion of a lift, referred to as the "positive," and the lowering motion, called the "negative," should be performed slowly, in a controlled fashion. That way, you effectively isolate the muscles being worked. Fast, jerky repetitions, on the other hand, don't isolate muscles but instead place harmful stress on the joints, ligaments, and tendons. Not only is this an unproductive way to tone muscles, it's also a dangerous training habit to adopt because it increases your risk of injury.

  At the midpoint or top of the exercise, pause for a second

to tense your muscles. Then lower the weight slowly again, accentuating the negative portion of the lift. Your muscles thus get maximum stimulation from the exercise.

- **Number of repetitions and sets.** Higher repetitions (12 or more) performed with moderate to heavy poundages help put your body in a fat-burning mode. So does performing more sets (series of repetitions). Increasing the number of sets uses up more calories, thus burning fat and increasing muscle tone.

The Workout Sequence

Between each set, immediately perform the designated fascial stretch for that set. (Refer to the workouts below.) The combination of exercise and stretching keeps you moving for better conditioning. This portion of the workout should take only thirty minutes.

Follow the strength-training/stretching portion of your workout with thirty to forty-five minutes of aerobics. By including aerobics in your routine, you more than double your fatburning power.

Workout Frequency

For best results, perform the Anticellulite Workout two to three times a week. Three times weekly, on nonconsecutive days, is preferable, particularly if you need to lose body fat. But if you just need to tighten up the muscles and skin on your lower body, twice a week is fine.

On non-stretch training days, try to work in one or two extra aerobic sessions. It's generally recognized that the best advances (especially in terms of fat loss) are made by four to five days of aerobics a week.

As noted earlier, each of your extra aerobic sessions should last at least thirty to forty-five minutes. Gradually try to work up to sixty minutes. The longer you do aerobics, the more fat you'll burn. After twenty minutes, your body starts relying more on fat for fuel, especially if you're working out in the upper end of your target zone. So for fat loss, you must try to work out aerobically for longer than twenty minutes.

Try to concentrate on upping your aerobic intensity too. For optimum fat-burning, you should exercise at a level hard enough to raise your heart rate 65 to 85 percent of your maximum heart rate (MHR), which is expressed as 220 minus your age.

Workout Choice

You can select from the two Anticellulite Workouts listed, or alternate them from workout to workout. On Tuesday, for example, you might do Workout #1; on Friday, Workout #2. You can mix and match your choices, just as long as you fit in at least two workouts a week.

The Anticellulite Workout targets thighs, hips, and buttocks exclusively. To firm up other portions of your body, you may want to perform some strength-training exercises for your upper body after working your lower body. Or you may opt to work your upper body on different workout days.

THE ANTICELLULITE WORKOUT
(Perform two to three times a week.)

WORKOUT #1

Warm-up: 5 minutes of moderate-intensity walking

Exercise Style: Moderate to heavy poundages with high repetitions (12–15)

Routine

Exercise	Sets	Repetitions
Barbell squat	Warm-up set (light weight) 2—increase poundage each set	10–12 12–15
Hip stretch	*3—perform between barbell squat sets*	*Hold stretch 10–20 seconds*
Leg extensions	Warm-up set (light weight) 2—increase poundage each set	10–12 12–15
Thigh stretch	*3—perform between leg extension sets*	*Hold stretch 10–20 seconds*
Leg curls	Warm-up set (light weight) 2—increase poundage each set	10–12 12–15
Forward hamstring stretch	*3—perform between leg extension sets*	*Hold stretch 10–20 seconds*
Walking dumb-bell lunges	Walk for 5 minutes, performing lunges.	As many as possible
Thigh stretch	*1 set performed after walking dumbbell lunges*	*Hold stretch 10–20 seconds*
Incline back kick	1 set	15–25
Forward hamstring stretch	*1 set performed after incline back kick*	*Hold stretch 10–20 seconds*
Cellulite burner	1 set	Perform as many repetitions as possible
Inner thigh stretch	*1 set performed after cellulite burner*	*Hold stretch 10–20 seconds*

Aerobics

Follow the above exercise routine with 30–45 minutes of aerobic exercise.

WORKOUT #2

Warm-up: 5–10 minutes of relaxed walking

Exercise Style: Moderate to heavy poundages with high repetitions (12–15)

Routine

Exercise	Sets	Repetitions
Freehand squat	3	12–15
Thigh stretch	*3—perform between freehand squat sets*	*Hold stretch 10–20 seconds*
Straight-leg deadlift	Warm-up set (light weight) 2—increase poundage each set	10–12 12–15
Butterfly	*3—perform between straight-leg deadlift sets*	*Hold stretch 10–20 seconds*
Side lunge	1	12–15 each leg
Inner/thigh hamstring stretch	*1—performed after side lunges*	*Hold stretch 10–20 seconds*
Walking dumb-bell lunges	Walk for 5 minutes, performing lunges	As many repetitions as possible
Hip stretch	*1—performed after walking lunges*	*Hold stretch 10–20 seconds*
Hip/hamstring curl or dumbbell buttocks burner	Warm-up set (light weight) 2—increase poundage each set	10–12 12–15
Forward hamstring stretch	*3—perform between hip/hamstring curl or dumbbell buttocks burner*	*Hold stretch 10–20 seconds*
Cellulite burner	1	As many repetitions as possible
Inner thigh stretch	*1—performed after cellulite burner*	*Hold stretch 10–20 seconds*

Aerobics

Follow the above exercise routine with 30–45 minutes of aerobic exercise

EXERCISE SUBSTITUTIONS

You may need to substitute exercises if you work out at home or if a certain machine indicated for your routine is not available at your workout facility. Or you may want to vary your routine by trying a different exercise every so often. The chart below provides a list of exercises that can be interchanged. For example, suppose your workout calls for leg extensions, but you don't have access to this equipment. Refer to the chart, and you'll see that a freehand squat can be substituted instead.

Anticellulite Exercises

Free Weights/ Generic	Machine	Nonapparatus
Barbell squat	Leg extensions	Freehand squat
Straight-leg deadlift	Leg curls	Walking dumbbell lunges without weight
Incline back kick	Hip/hamstring curl	Walking dumbbell lunges without weight; or back kick lying on floor or mat
Dumbbell buttocks burner	Hip/hamstring curl	Lunges, any type, using a weighted object such as a heavy book
Cellulite burner	Leg curl, or hip/ hamstring curl	Lunges, any type, using a weighted object such as a heavy book

PART V

SUPPORTIVE TREATMENTS

CHAPTER 13

Endermologie Against Cellulite

Do you have to bare your thighs any time soon? Then consider a cellulite-minimizing procedure called Endermologie. It is an innovative form of deep massage that has been shown in scientific studies to reduce the appearance of cellulite, reshape the body, increase skin elasticity, and temporarily trim the circumference of the thighs. Endermologie may also improve the appearance of stretch marks and tighten up loose skin.

What Is Endermologie?

Endermologie was developed in the 1970s in France by an engineer named Louis Paul Guitay, who had been severely burned in a car accident. Part of his recovery involved morning and afternoon manual massage sessions by a physical therapist. The goal of therapy was to soften the scars resulting from the accident.

Guitay noticed that the afternoon sessions were not as effective as those given in the morning, because the therapist's hands and strokes were considerably weaker due to fatigue. In response, he invented a special mechanical machine that could be used in place of manual massage to treat burn victims and thus ease therapist fatigue. Guitay dubbed the machine and the procedure "Endermologie," derived from *ende*, meaning "under," and *derm*, for "skin." The procedure was widely used to soften scars and to standardize therapeutic massage techniques.

The massager, which is handheld and makes a sucking noise, vaguely resembles a pasta machine. Attached to a larger machine via a suction hose, the unit works by lifting and drawing the skin into a fold between two motorized rollers. The action of rollers kneads and massages the skin. The massager has programmable strength and speed settings.

Although the device was originally intended for physical therapy, French therapists noticed that it ironed out the dimpled skin on women's legs and improved overall body contour. They began using the machines for cellulite reduction, and the treatment became wildly popular throughout Europe, where it now is as routine as getting your hair or nails done.

Endermologie was introduced to the United States in 1996 for use by physicians and technicians for treating cellulite. Within a year of its introduction, approximately three hundred board-certified plastic surgeons in the United States had acquired machines. More than twice that many employ the procedure today.

The machines are manufactured and marketed by a French company named LPG Endermologie, which has a U.S. subsidiary, LPG USA. In 1998, LPG USA received clearance from the FDA to use the massager and the procedure to treat cellulite. By law, the company is allowed to claim that the machine results in "temporary reduction in the appearance of cellulite."

How Does Endermologie Work?

Its massaging action has at least three benefits. First, it increases blood and lymph circulation in the fat layer, releasing and eliminating any accumulated wastes and toxins. Improved circulation may also assist in fat burning. Water is evacuated from connective tissue too, reducing limb girth and contributing to a thinner appearance.

Second, the massaging action stretches and softens connective tissue to improve outer skin quality and texture. The net effect is a smoother, less dimply appearance.

Third, Endermologie may stimulate special cells called fibroblasts. These are the mother cells of connective tissue; they give birth to new collagen and elastin. Their stimulation by Endermologie may renew collagen and elastic production, rejuvenate underlying tissue, and thus promote skin elasticity.

In a study of women conducted at Southwest Texas State University, those who completed a series of at least seven Endermologie treatments showed an average loss in body diameter (after measuring waist, hip, thigh, knee, and calf) of 0.5 inches (1.38 centimeters). Those who finished fourteen treatments trimmed their body diameter by as much as 1.12 inches (2.85 centimeters) on average.

In a second study conducted by the same researchers, women who underwent seven Endermologie treatments pared their body diameter by 0.5 inches (1.34 centimeters); those treated with fourteen treatments reduced their body diameter by 0.72 inches (1.83 centimeters).

In another study, in which Endermologie was performed five days a week for one month, the procedure pared thigh girth ever so slightly: by only 0.07 inches (1.85 millimeters) after the twelfth treatment, and by 0.20 inches (4.98 millimeters) after the twentieth treatment. Clearly, Endermologie reduces measurements, if only temporarily, but results vary widely among women.

Research conducted on Yucatan minipigs at the Vanderbilt University School of Medicine in Nashville demonstrated that Endermologie noticeably smoothes out cellulite. (The skin of minipigs is similar to human skin—which is why these animals were used in the experiment.) The researchers believe that the technique relaxes the connective tissue holding fat cells in place. The reduced tension on these tissues created more room in the fat chambers, causing less fat to bulge out.

In a study at the University of Southern California, Los Angeles (UCLA), researchers discovered that Endermologie's massaging action quadrupled blood flow to the treated areas. Also significant: Five times more lymphatic fluid flowed away. These results hint that Endermologie is an effective way to treat two culprits in cellulite formation: poor circulation and sluggish lymph drainage.

What to Expect

Prior to your session, you'll be issued a nylon body suit to wear for sanitary reasons, but also to help the machine glide over your skin more easily. At most clinics, you'll sign a waiver acknowledging that the procedure provides no guaranteed results.

Endermologie is performed at plastic surgery clinics and skin-care salons. Estheticians at skin-care salons use it to treat mild cases of cellulite. If performed in a medical clinic, the procedure is usually supervised by a physician and is used to treat more advanced cases of cellulite.

A series of fifteen to twenty sessions, one or two a week, is recommended. Sessions usually last thirty minutes to an hour. During the session, the technician focuses on cellulite-affected areas, but massages other areas as well to stimulate general circulation and internal cleansing.

Monthly follow-up sessions are advisable too, since cellulite can return. Each treatment costs between $70 and $100; some clinics offer package deals.

While undergoing treatment, you should adhere to some additional instructions:

- Drink eight to ten glasses of water daily. Water helps flush toxins from your system.
- Follow a low-fat diet.
- Exercise regularly to strengthen leg muscles.

These practices optimize the results you get from Endermologie. The ideal candidates are less than thirty pounds overweight, ages thirty to forty-five, exercise regularly, and are in generally good health.

What About Side Effects?

Endermologie is a nonsurgical, noninvasive procedure, so it is relatively painless and leaves no soreness. Some people complain of discomfort and bruising, but only after the first few treatments.

Other clients have no problems at all—and begin to see results after just three or four treatments. Most women who undergo Endermologie are pleased with the results and say their legs feel firmer and their clothes looser. Others say their "saddlebags" disappear with treatment. Your friends may ask you if you've lost weight, because you'll look slimmer in all the right places. In fact, weight loss is often a pleasant side effect of Endermologie. The procedure is catching on with men too, who like the difference it makes in reducing love handles.

Endermologie is also being used to accelerate and improve healing following liposuction. Writing in the medical journal *Aesthetic Plastic Surgery,* Peter Bela Fodor, M.D., observed: "I have used the LPG intraoperatively (just after liposuction) on more than 20 patients over the last two months. An impressive reduction of postoperative edema and ecchymosis [bruising] as early as two to three days after surgery was noted and documented with standardized photography."

Used in conjunction with liposuction, Endermologie is also thought to evenly redistribute remaining fat cells and improve blood flow.

Where to Find an Endermologie Clinic

Endermologie clinics are springing up everywhere—in the offices of plastic surgeons, in skin-care clinics, at retail malls, and in day spas. To locate an establishment near you, refer to your local Yellow Pages, or call plastic surgery clinics or skin-care salons in your area to check availability.

Another excellent resource is the Web site www.cellulite usa.com. It lists the names, addresses, and phone numbers of Endermologie clinics in the United States, Canada, and United Kingdom that choose to advertise on the site. You'll find numerous clinics listed by state, province, or country.

Other Forms of Anticellulite Massage

THE SILKLIGHT THERAPEUTIC MASSAGE DEVICE

The SilkLight Therapeutic Massage Device is another massager that temporarily reduces the appearance of cellulite and improves body tone. It works in a manner similar to Endermologie, with a series of rolling and suction motions that mechanically manipulate subcutaneous layers of fat. The massaging action improves blood circulation and lymphatic activity. It also relieves muscle tension.

With SilkLight, you can expect to see improvement in cellulite-affected skin after fourteen to seventeen sessions. Follow-up treatments are recommended to maintain skin smoothness. Physicians who employ the SilkLight say that it is capable of temporarily reducing body size by a combined average of eight inches from the arms, buttocks, hips, and thighs.

The SilkLight Therapeutic Massage Device system was developed by ESC Medical Systems Ltd., a company headquartered in Israel that manufactures and markets medical devices for the treatment of varicose veins, hair removal, skin cancer, skin rejuvenation, and other aesthetic applications. The company also markets surgical lasers for a wide range of medical applications.

LYMPHATIC MASSAGE

This type of massage is usually performed by trained physical or occupational therapists. Limbs are massaged in the direction of blood flow to unblock the lymphatic system and help promote lymph drainage. This leads to reduced swelling in the tissues. A single massage session takes approximately one hour and is recommended three times a week.

Cancer and surgical patients suffering from lymphedema are usually candidates for lymphatic massage, although other patients may be referred to therapy by their physicians.

HOME MASSAGERS

Various companies are now manufacturing and marketing do-it-yourself massagers designed to treat cellulite in the comfort of your own home—no need to go to a clinic or day spa. One of these is a massager called Cellesse, made by Philips. It lifts the skin by suction, and draws it between two rollers. All it takes is fifteen to twenty minutes on each leg, three times a week. You may see noticeable results in about a month. The device costs about $300. It should not be used if you have varicose veins, scars, or irritated skin, or if you are suffering from a heart condition, diabetes, blood circulation disease, or other medical problem. For more information on Cellese, go to www.edmart.com.

Another device is the IGIÁ Cellulift Massage System. Designed to temporarily improve cellulite, this massager uses a combination of massage, heat, and suction. It costs between $100 and $129 and can be ordered through the Web site www.vendusa.com/cellulift.htm.

CELLULITE STICK

This product is a nineteen-inch stick with a special center core designed to be vigorously rubbed across cellulite-prone areas. Recommended usage is two to three sessions a day, five minutes each time. Promotional literature on the product states that it works to temporarily reduce the appearance of cellulite in two ways: by increasing tissue temperature to promote the burning of accumulated fat cells and by unlocking the connective tissue responsible for dimpling.

The Cellulite Stick is manufactured and marketed by Cellulite Rx. For more information on the product and pricing, call 1–800–987–7845, or access the company's Web site at www. Cellulite-Rx.com.

DRY SKIN BRUSHING

Dry skin brushing is a technique that increases blood and lymph circulation to cellulite-affected areas, plus improves skin texture and appearance. With a stiff brush or massage glove, brush your skin in an upward direction—from your feet toward your heart. Use gentle strokes, and avoid brushing over any skin wounds or sores. Try to brush every day for about five to ten minutes. After dry skin brushing, apply an anticellulite cream to your thighs. The improved blood circulation and lymph drainage from dry skin brushing is believed to enhance the therapeutic effect of the cream.

SHIATSU

This traditional form of Japanese massage has been used to treat cellulite, although infrequently. With shiatsu, the therapist applies firm finger pressure to specific points on the body to balance energy flow. You lie on a padded surface or floor— no massage table—and the therapist kneels next to you. Shiatsu is normally used to treat lower back pain, nervous disorders, and other ailments. It also helps relieve constipation, a factor in the development of cellulite.

CHAPTER 14

Anticellulite Creams and Lotions

As we search for ways to eradicate cellulite, products called thigh creams promise to do it for us. Just slather them over the cellulite-affected skin and eventually the cottage cheese look will be a thing of the past. Or so the products claim.

But can you truly find help in a jar or a bottle?

To some degree, yes. Topical creams may minimize the appearance of cellulite, but will not dissolve or remove it. If powerful enough to do so, they would also dissolve skin, muscles, and other body tissues. There is, however, some interesting clinical evidence demonstrating that these products can somehow reduce the girth of the thighs and improve the appearance of cellulite-affected skin.

Available in creams, lotions, gels, or spray formulas, hundreds of thigh-slimming products are now on the market. They go by various names: thigh creams, skin-firming lotions, and body-contouring formulas, to name just a few. For the cosmetics industry, these products represent a $200 million a year market. You can purchase them over the counter at pharmacies, department stores, mass merchandisers, boutiques, and spas.

From pharmaceuticals to herbs, there are a wide variety of ingredients in these products. All are designed to be rubbed into the skin, and claim to work by various mechanisms. As a consumer, you should be familiar with these products, what they contain, and what they can and cannot do for cellulite.

Methylxanthines

Methylxanthines are a group of drugs that have been touted for their fat-burning action. They include aminophylline, theophylline (a chemical cousin of aminophylline), and caffeine. All have been shown to break down fat in test tube experiments. Caffeine, in particular, promotes the production of adrenaline, a hormone that accelerates the release of fatty acids into the bloodstream. It also stimulates the metabolism and is rapidly absorbed by the body when applied as part of a topical formulation.

Perhaps the best known of the anticellulite methylxanthines is aminophylline, widely advertised as a cosmetic that removes cellulite from the skin. There are approximately sixty thigh cream products, containing concentrations ranging from 0.5 to 2 percent aminophylline.

Aminophylline is an approved oral antihistamine drug used in some asthma medications. It relaxes the smooth muscles of the respiratory tract. Taken internally, aminophylline also acts as a diuretic, drawing water from cells. Like caffeine, aminophylline helps liberate fatty acids and release them into the bloodstream. It easily penetrates the outer layer of the skin when applied topically.

Aminophylline stepped into the spotlight in 1994, when two researchers reported the results of a small study conducted with eleven women who used a cream containing the drug. Five days a week for six weeks, they applied a 2 percent aminophylline cream to one thigh and a nonaminophylline cream (the placebo) to the other. By the end of the experimental period, the aminophylline cream had reduced the size of the women's treated thighs from 0.28 inches (0.7 centimeters) to 0.9 inches (2.3 centimeters), and left those thighs looking smoother.

In another study, the results were similar: Five overweight women applied aminophylline cream daily to one thigh, and a placebo cream to the other. After four weeks, the range of reductions in thigh circumference reported by the researchers was 0.28 inches (0.73 centimeters) to 0.89 inches (2.27 centimeters).

Both studies concluded that aminophylline cream produces targeted fat loss if applied topically to the thighs for four to six weeks. In other words, it tricks the body into giving up hard-to-budge thigh fat.

As an anticellulite agent, the drug is believed to work by affecting a hormone called phosphodiesterase, which is abundant in women's thighs and hips and equally abundant in men's bellies. Phosphodiesterase blocks the messenger in charge of releasing fat from fat cells. Aminophylline steps in and interferes with the action of phosphodiesterase, clearing the way for fat breakdown. Fat molecules can then be dismantled into fatty acids, released into the bloodstream, and ultimately burned for energy. Aminophylline may also shrink fat cells.

Aminophylline is steeped in controversy, however. Not all scientists are convinced that it can trigger these fat-burning events, even though fat cells in test tubes do give up fat when mixed with aminophylline. Further, one possible explanation for the reduction in thigh girth and improvement in appearance may be water loss, since aminophylline is a diuretic.

As with many such agents, aminophylline does not work for everyone. Several years ago, I tried a jar of aminophylline-based cream as part of a televised experiment. A local television reporter asked me to apply the cream to the back of my thighs for six weeks. I complied, and following the experimental period, my "before and after" photos were bared on the nightly news. Unfortunately, no discernible difference could be seen in my thighs.

Aminophylline thigh creams seem to have no adverse side

effects. A study conducted in 1994 analyzed the blood chemistries of 702 women, half of whom used the active cream and the other half a placebo cream. No significant changes were found in blood cell counts, cholesterol levels, or other test variables. Approximately 2 percent of the subjects were allergic to the cream. Allergic symptoms included redness, itching, and blisterlike reactions. Another study looked into the effect of a 2 percent aminophylline-based cream on heart rate and pulmonary function, but found no untoward reactions.

Jars of aminophylline creams cost about $40 on average. Even though some clinical research backs up their benefit, further studies are needed on topical creams containing methylxanthines, including their long-term health effects. It is important to note that you must continue using the cream to maintain its benefits.

Thiomucase

Thiomucase is an enzyme derived from the testicles of bulls that is used in numerous therapeutic applications, including the treatment of scars and in cellulite reduction. Thiomucase acts on fibrous components of connective tissue called mucopolysaccharides that are found in cellulite tissue, as well as in scar tissue. This enzyme breaks up mucopolysaccharide fibers to improve blood flow to the tissue and help remove cellulite.

Thiomucase is available in a product called Thiomucase Creme, often used by bodybuilders and other athletes because it visibly tightens the skin and may reduce signs of aging.

Topical Herbals

Numerous cosmetics companies formulate their anticellulite creams with mixtures of herbal extracts. In addition, a number of spa treatments are available that combine heat, massage, and pastes of herbal extracts applied to the thighs and buttocks. Among the extracts found in herbal-based thigh creams and wraps are the following:

Algae. Algae are a group of aquatic plants that include kelp, bladderwrack, and other forms of seaweed. All are believed to exert a range of healing effects. Algae are rich in iodine, a mineral required by the body in tiny amounts and essential for the healthy functioning of the thyroid gland. The thyroid gland sets the pace at which metabolism occurs.

Algae are also said to improve circulation in the tissues and promote a general firming across the outermost layer of the skin when applied topically.

Barley. Barley is a grain normally used to provide nutrition to the body. Taken orally as a tea or soup, it is a folk medicine used to treat stomach disorders. When applied topically, barley may stimulate circulation to the tissues and improve lymphatic drainage. (Circulation and lymphatic drainage are believed to be sluggish in women with cellulite.)

Birch bark. Birch bark contains a chemical called methyl salicylate that is similar to aspirin. When applied topically, birch bark decreases inflammation, which may be why it is used in anticellulite creams. (One theory holds that cellulite formation is caused by inflammation.) Birch bark is also an astringent that creates a temporary tightening effect when applied to the skin.

Butcher's broom. Derived from an evergreen shrub that grows in Europe, the roots and rhizome of this plant are used orally as a circulatory tonic and an antiinflammatory agent. Butchers once used the plant's leaves to scrub their chopping blocks, hence the name. Like birch bark, butcher's broom is an astringent that temporarily tightens the skin when applied topically.

Cangzhu root. This herbal extract is a chief ingredient in Clarins Body Lift 2000, a cellulite-fighting product. In tests, Body Lift trimmed thigh girth by an average of one inch in 85 percent of the subjects. The product reduced the thickness of the fatty layer by up to 25 percent and improved skin firmness by up to 45 percent. These improvements occurred after only thirty days of use.

Cassava. Better known as tapioca, cassava is a widely cultivated root crop grown for food around the world. It is believed to trigger an enzyme that helps pull sugars and fats from cells.

Elderberry. Elderberry supposedly helps reduce water retention when applied topically.

Fennel. Fennel is an herb used medicinally, as well as in cooking. It has no known weight loss benefits, but is generally regarded as safe. Fennel oil is sometimes used as massage lubricant.

Fenugreek. The seeds of the fenugreek plant yield a skin-softening oil used in body-care products.

Forskolin. Derived from the roots of the plant *Coleus forskohlii*, this herb has been used to treat asthma and may have properties similar to aminophylline. Forskolin has been used in Indian medicine for centuries to treat a wide range of ailments.

Ginkgo Biloba. *Ginkgo biloba*, derived from the leaves of an ornamental tree, improves blood circulation to the skin. It is used both as a topical and an oral treatment for cellulite.

Guarana. Guarana is a red berry from a plant grown in the Amazon Valley. It contains seven times as much caffeine as the coffee bean and is widely sold in health food stores as an oral supplement to increase energy. The supplement is made from the seeds of the berry. The caffeine-rich guarana extract has been used in some thigh creams as a slimming agent.

Hazelnut. The oil of the hazelnut is thought to reduce fluid retention when applied topically. It also acts as a skin lubricant and helps the skin maintain elasticity.

Hawkweed. Hawkweed grows wild in Europe and in the prairies and woodlands of the northwestern U.S. It was named hawkweed because the ancient Greeks imagined that hawks used the plant to strengthen their eyesight. In folk medicine, hawkweed has had many uses. The herb is said to help tissue drainage and stimulate blood circulation.

Horse chestnut. Seeds of the horse chestnut plant are processed into extracts used orally to treat chronic venous insufficiency and swelling in the legs. Topical application is believed to improve circulation and reduce swelling. One of the herb's active ingredients, aescin, is used in some oral anticellulite supplements. Aescin inhibits vein swelling, strengthens and tones blood vessels, and works as an antiinflammatory agent.

Ivy. Ivy is a member of the ginseng family and shares some of its health benefits, namely improved tissue drainage and blood flow.

Japanese green tea. Green tea contains caffeine, a methylxanthine that may exert a fat-burning effect, and is plentiful in other health-building chemicals.

Kola nut. Kola nut is a caffeine-containing herb used in many anticellulite creams and lotions. It is described as a lipolytic (fat burner) in the German Commission E monographs.

Lemon. The juice of the lemon is an astringent that tightens the skin when applied topically. Extracts of citrus fruits also moisturize the skin.

Marjoram. A member of the mint family, marjoram is an ancient healing herb with mild antiseptic properties. It is also used to flavor a variety of foods. Marjoram is said to promote perspiration and thus may combat fluid retention in the tissues.

Rosemary. Rosemary is a multitalented herb, used down through the ages to treat many types of ailments, probably because it contains antioxidants known to protect the immune system.

Rosemary is a popular ingredient in many cosmetics, including wrinkle creams, moisturizers, hair tonics, and shampoos.

Rutin. An extract of citrus fruits, rutin is believed to prevent excess carbohydrates from being metabolized into storage fat.

Sesame oil. Oil extracted from sesame seeds yields a moisturizing lubricant that is used in many cosmetics.

Shea butter. A relatively new ingredient finding its way into cosmetics, shea comes from the seed of an African tree that is related to the coconut. Shea butter, or oil, is water-soluble and acts as a moisturizer.

Strawberry. Strawberry is an astringent that may temporarily tighten the skin when applied topically.

Sweet clover. Applied externally, sweet clover reduces fluid buildup caused by inflammation and improves lymph drainage.

Yerba maté. Yerba maté is a South American plant whose leaves are dried and made into tea, put into capsules, or formulated for topical use in skin-firming cosmetics. Yerba maté contains the highest natural concentration of theophylline and caffeine of any herb.

Yohimbe. Yohimbe is an herb derived from the bark of an evergreen grown in West Africa. It is best known for its aphrodisiac properties, because it stimulates erection. One of its active ingredients is yohimbine. Yohimbine stimulates the release of noradrenaline (norepinephrine), a hormone that raises body temperature and helps liberate fatty acids from cells to be burned as fuel.

The Evidence for Topical Herbals

Can products formulated with mixtures of herbal extracts downsize your thighs? A couple of studies say *yes*. However, the reductions range from slight to moderate.

In 1996, a group of researchers published the results of a study testing the fat-reduction power of an herbal cream containing caffeine, horse chestnut, ivy, algae, bladderwrack, plankton (an alga), butcher's broom, and soy protein. Subjects applied the cream to their thighs for thirty days.

By the end of the experimental period, subcutaneous fat had decreased in thickness by 0.11 inches (2.8 millimeters) on average, as measured by ultrasound. But the fatty layer returned to its prior thickness once the cream application had been discontinued. The researchers theorized that the cream somehow made the fat cells more compact, but could not explain reasons for the relapse in the size of the fatty layer.

In clinical research, Vichy Laboratories, a division of L'Oreal, tested its anticellulite product, Glucoblock, with positive results. Women reduced the circumference of their upper thighs by 0.75 inches (1.9 centimeters) in an average of twenty-eight days and lost at least one grade of orange-peel appearance on their skin as determined by a group of doctors involved as observers in the study. Further, 91 percent of the women who used the product thought their clothes fit more loosely. Glucoblock contains aescin, gingko, caffeine, and salicyclic acid.

It is clear that topical herbal slimming products do some good, if only temporarily. Most contain a smart dose of ingredients that seem to firm up sagging skin and smooth out cellulite. Some appear to downsize thigh diameter. They do not work for everyone, however. Even so, there is certainly no harm in trying them, particularly since they appear to provide a quick fix for cellulite.

Using Thigh Creams

Thigh creams are usually applied to the specific areas at least twice a day. You should follow the manufacturer's recommended application schedule, however. These products range in cost from $40 to $185 per bottle or jar.

Other Products with Promise

RETINOIDS

Quite probably, you know retinoids best as the nutritional supplements vitamin A and beta-carotene, or the acne and antiwrinkle medications Retin-A and Renova, also known generically as tretinoin or retinoic acid.

Retinoids, particularly Retin-A, have been evaluated as

potential cellulite fighters. Some investigators have theorized that cellulite develops as the skin loses its firmness and elasticity. Retin-A stimulates the formation of collagen, the protein that keeps your skin firm. Retin-A also thickens the top layer (the epidermis) of your skin, making it look more compact. New blood vessels form in the epidermis too, for improved blood flow. All of these actions would be beneficial in treating cellulite, but to date no large-scale studies have been conducted on retinoids as anticellulite agents.

There are certain side effects associated with Retin-A usage. According to the *Physicians' Desk Reference*, Retin-A may make your skin overly sensitive to sun, and it could become severely sunburned if exposed to daylight. In some people, skin irritation may occur with use.

COENZYME Q10 CREAMS

Technically known as ubiquinone, coenzyme Q10 (abbreviated as CoQ10) is a nutrient found naturally inside the mitochondria of the cell, where it is involved in the conversion of food to energy. It also acts as an antioxidant, capable of disarming free radicals.

As an oral supplement, coenzyme Q10 has many health-giving properties. For example, it helps improve cardiac function, strengthens the immune system, and may enhance the quality of overall health.

Coenzyme Q10 is also a key constituent of certain skin creams. These products are designed to counter photoaging—the skin changes that take place over time from long-term exposure to the sun. Skin wrinkling is the best-known effect of photoaging, but cellulite is thought to be an end result too.

Prolonged sun exposure activates an enzyme called collagenase that breaks down collagen, the main structural protein in connective tissue. The normally elastic fibers in the skin begin to degenerate over time, leading to sagging, wrinkled skin. Sun exposure also increases free radicals, which are another possible culprit in cellulite formation.

A recent study found that topical application of coenzyme Q10 has the power to prevent many of the effects of photoaging. The nutrient reduced wrinkle depth, suppressed free radical damage, and interfered with the destructive action of collagenase. This is certainly good news for anyone with prematurely aged skin.

Coenzyme Q10 creams are marketed primarily for the treatment of facial wrinkles. Although it's too early to tell, these creams may be of value in treating cellulite-ridden skin, since they appear to prevent structural skin damage.

LACTIC ACID

Lactic acid, glycolic acid, and other alpha-hydroxy acids are derived from fruits and vegetables. Lactic acid has been mentioned in medical literature as a possible anticellulite agent. It exfoliates dead skin cells from the stratum corneum—a layer on the surface of the epidermis—and improves its condition. In doing so, the appearance of cellulite is somewhat minimized, with less bumpiness. Further, lactic acid has been shown in research to firm, thicken, and smooth out facial skin.

Treating the skin with glycolic acid has been shown in scientific experiments to generate tissue-producing fibroblasts, accelerate the production of collagen, and reverse sun-related skin aging. These findings hold promise not only for antiaging treatments, but also for anticellulite treatments.

Several anticellulite creams on the market contain fruit and vegetable acids. However, there are not yet any published studies showing that lactic acid or other alpha-hydroxy acids can specifically treat cellulite.

SELF-TANNERS

An excellent way to camouflage cellulite—and still bare your legs—is to apply a self-tanner. A darker skin color will even out your skin tone, plus reduce the shadows caused by skin puckering. Self-tanners are generally safe for most skin types. Some contain sunscreens for protection against ultraviolet rays, believed to be responsible for breaking down collagen and further aggravating cellulite.

The Five-Step Cellulite Cure

It's encouraging to know that cellulite can be treated successfully with natural therapies, and that you *can* develop a more
youthful, cellulite-resistant body. You don't need expensive
cosmetic surgery, either. All it takes is knowledge and commitment to keep yourself healthy, attractive, and cellulite resistant. Let's review the five steps of the Cellulite Breakthrough
Plan:

**Step 1.   Consider the use of nutritional supplements,
including cellulite control supplements, natural fat
burners, antioxidants, calcium, energy bars and
drinks, and fiber supplements.**

**Step 2.   Follow a healthy, cellulite-fighting diet, as out-
lined in chapters 7 and 8. These nutritional principles are incorporated in the 30-Day Anticellulite
Diet.**

Step 3. **Exercise regularly, using a combination of strength training, fascial stretching, and aerobics.**

Step 4. **Optimize your results from supplementation, diet, and exercise by using supportive treatments such as massage and anticellulite creams.**

Step 5. **Maintain a cellulite-resistant body by making permanent changes in your lifestyle.**

This last step is probably the most important. The total plan for minimizing and eliminating cellulite embraces not one but every facet of your life. It includes nutrition, exercise, respect for your body, and a positive attitude.

Making lifestyle changes in these areas requires day-by-day determination and commitment. Every moment you make one healthy choice is a success, and each choice makes the next one easier. Continue to make changes, until healthy habits have become ingrained in your life. Before long, you'll begin to experience a fitness you can see and feel. You will not want to return to your former life, with its less-than-desirable habits!

Nutritionally, you don't have to be a purist 100 percent of the time. Have some splurges every now and then, and don't feel guilty about them.

But be a purist when it comes to exercising. Keep moving and keep working out! If the body doesn't move, its supporting structures like muscles, connective tissue, and bones start *degenerating*. The exercising body, on the other hand, is *regenerating* itself, especially with the right nutrients providing the raw material for growth, maintenance, and lifelong health and vitality.

The main purpose of this book has been to teach you how to minimize, even eliminate, cellulite, but it's really about getting and staying healthy. If you do all that's required, then having—and keeping—a cellulite-resistant body is just one of many pleasant side effects.

As I've already pointed out, there are numerous health benefits to this program, such as reduced risk for disease, higher energy levels, and a more physically fit body. By changing your lifestyle permanently—and for the better—you'll put yourself on the path to active, lifelong health.

APPENDIX A

Should You Consider Liposuction?

Among cosmetic surgeries performed in the United States, the most common is liposuction to reduce thigh size, according to the American Society of Plastic and Reconstructive Surgeons (ASPRS). Liposuction is a shaping procedure in which unwanted fat is removed from specific sections of the body, including the abdomen, hips, buttocks, thighs, knees, upper arms, chin, cheeks, and neck.

Contrary to popular belief, liposuction is not designed to treat cellulite, but rather to remove stubborn, deep-layer fat deposits that do not respond well to dieting. During liposuction, a surgeon normally spares the subcutaneous fat layer in which cellulite is found in order to preserve its network of blood and lymph vessels and to provide a smoother body contour after the operation. Some surgeons, however, do try to treat cellulite with liposuction of the subcutaneous fat layer, but this approach has not been universally successful.

In truth, liposuction may make cellulite worse. Writing in the October 1996 issue of *Clinics in Plastic Surgery,* Ted Lockwood, M.D., observed: "The most common long-term aesthetic complication of liposuction is skin laxity with surface contour irregularities (cellulite), resulting in an acceleration of the aged appearance of the skin."

In other words, liposuction can make your skin looser and more cellulite-ridden, plus it may further age your skin. Clearly, cellulite responds best to natural—not surgical—solutions.

If considering liposuction, you must approach it with reasonable expectations: as a procedure to remove hard-to-budge fat and recontour your figure, not to eliminate cellulite. If fat removal and body recontouring are your goals, here is a closer look at what you need to know about liposuction, including its risks.

The Best Candidates for Liposuction

To be a good candidate for liposuction, you must also meet certain criteria. The best candidate for liposuction:

- **Exhibits general good health.** Your surgeon will take a careful medical history, looking for such prior complications as vein clotting, and circulatory problems, blood disorders, evidence of smoking (smoking increases the risk of abnormal blood clotting), hypertension; and other medical problems that may adversely affect healing.

   In addition, your surgeon will probably ask you about any medications you're taking. Aspirin, alcohol, warfarin (Coumadin), vitamin E, and vitamin E–containing products may increase bleeding during surgery. Thus, it's wise to avoid these products for a few weeks prior to your operation.
- **Has firm, elastic skin.** Elastic skin will retract better following surgery than aging skin will.
- **Is relatively young (less than forty years old).** Older patients generally have less skin elasticity and may not achieve the same results as a younger woman with tighter skin.
- **Is not obese or substantially overweight.** Liposuction is not a substitute for weight loss. In fact, the procedure results in only the loss of two to four pounds, on average. Writing in the journal *Medical Clinics of North America*, four medical authorities observed: "Because human adipose [fat] tissue is distributed so widely in subcutaneous and deeper depots, it is difficult to make a major inroad on human obesity by surgical methods."

   The best candidates for liposuction are women whose weight is stable or who are at their ideal weight. Many women find that having liposuction makes it easier to maintain their weight and stay motivated to do so.

- **Can afford the procedure.** Liposuction is not cheap, ranging from $1,000 to $5,000 or more, depending on the number of sites treated. According to the ASPR, the average surgeon's fee for liposuction in 1998 was $1,872 for each single site. For a technique known as ultrasound-assisted liposuction (explained on p. 216), the average fee was $3,827 for each single site. Liposuction is generally not covered by health insurance, because it is an elective cosmetic procedure.

- **Is psychologically stable.** If you're undertaking any type of plastic surgery, you should be doing so to please yourself, not to satisfy someone else, solve a life problem, or motivate people to treat you differently.

    A woman with a psychological disturbance such as depression is generally a poor candidate because she lacks the emotional strength to endure the physical and psychological stress of the surgery. Women with eating disorders do not make good candidates, either, because they have distorted body images and may not be satisfied with the final results of liposuction, no matter how pleasing or successful. Further, it is critical that you discuss with your surgeon what liposuction can and cannot achieve so that you have realistic expectations prior to surgery.

Liposuction Techniques

The first documented case of liposuction was performed in France in 1921, when a French surgeon used a uterine curette to extract fat from the knees and calves of a well-known dancer. Sadly, the dancer developed an infection and had to have the infected leg amputated.

In the 1950s and 1960s, surgeons made incisions in the body to remove fat and skin. Unsightly scars and bulging skin were frequent complications. In the late 1960s, a surgeon in Germany began to suction out fat and fluid using a vacuum pump. This technique was later refined during the 1970s and 1980s by doctors working simultaneously in various countries, including the United States. Today, there are various types of liposuction performed by plastic surgeons, and the surgery is still evolving.

Before considering the procedure, learn about the various types of liposuction and ask your plastic surgeon which one is best for you—and why.

In all forms of liposuction, the surgeon makes a tiny incision in one or more locally anesthetized areas of the body and inserts a narrow tube called a cannula into the incision. The cannula is pushed and pulled through the fat layer to break up fat cells and then suction them out. A vacuum pump or a large syringe provides the suction action.

Along with fat, fluid is removed too. This fluid must be replenished during the procedure to prevent shock. Accordingly, you may be given intravenous fluids during and after surgery. Liposuction generally lasts one to two hours.

Your plastic surgeon may use one of several technique variations, in addition to the basic liposuction method described above.

The most common and advanced technique is called tumescent liposuction. It involves injecting a solution of salt water, lidocaine (a local anesthetic), and epinephrine (a hormone that shrinks blood vessels) into the fat layer prior to the procedure. The solution facilitates the removal of fat, reduces blood loss, and numbs the tissue during and after surgery. It also reduces the amount of bruising after surgery. Because blood loss is reduced during tumescent liposuction, there is less need for a blood transfusion during the procedure. The use of large volumes of injected fluid decreases or eliminates the need for intravenous sedation and general anesthesia. Tumescent liposuction derives its name from the fact that the fatty tissues, when filled with solution, are tumesced, or swollen.

Once the solution is injected, a small incision is made in the skin and the cannula is inserted into the fatty layer. The fat is then suctioned out as described above.

Speaking at the American Academy of Dermatology's annual meeting in 1998, William P. Coleman III, M.D., cited the benefits of this popular procedure: "Its chief advantages are that liposuction can be performed on an ambulatory basis, patients feel good immediately after the procedure, are able to walk on their own, experience minimal bruising, and recovery is rapid."

A technique similar to tumescent liposuction is the super-wet technique. It uses less fluid, however. Usually, the amount of fluid injected matches the amount of fat to be removed.

Many plastic surgeons in the United States are using a relatively new technique called ultrasound-assisted lipoplasty (UAL). Performed in Europe and South America for nearly a decade, it involves the use of a special cannula, which generates high-frequency sound waves that liquefy fat cells. The cannula used to perform UAL is slightly larger than the type used for traditional liposuction, and longer skin incisions are therefore required.

During UAL, a fluid containing a local anesthetic is injected into the fatty layer, and the cannula is guided through the fat tissue. The ultrasonic energy explodes the walls of the fat cells, liquefying the fat. The liquefied fat and injected fluid are then removed using traditional liposuction techniques.

Because the fat is liquefied, more can be removed with UAL than with other forms of liposuction. In addition, there is usually less blood loss, bruising, and pain with UAL.

Some plastic surgeons feel that UAL may provide a surgical solution to cellulite removal because it can better extract fat from the sub-cutaneous layers. This potential benefit has not been proven conclusively, however. A 1997 study conducted by physicians Helena Igra, M.D., and Nancy M. Satur, M.D., looked into whether there are operative and cosmetic differences (including cellulite improvement) between tumescent liposuction and UAL. Twenty-eight people (twenty-five women and three men) participated in their study. Some of the volunteers underwent tumescent liposuction; the remainder, UAL.

An independent physician observer was employed to evaluate differences in the outcomes of the two procedures. In comparing the results from both procedures, the evaluating physician could detect no significant differences in the degree of postoperative swelling, skin retraction, or decreased cellulite.

Preparing for Liposuction

Prior to surgery, you will be photographed for a record of before-and-after results. You may also be asked to donate your own blood, in case it is needed during the procedure.

Quite probably, your surgeon will advise you to eat a well-balanced diet before and after surgery. It is important to increase your protein and calorie intake, since surgery increases those requirements enormously—by as much as 50 to 100 percent. You may also be instructed to supplement with additional vitamin C and iron. Vitamin C helps accelerate wound healing and reduces the degree of bruising. Iron aids in rebuilding red blood cells.

You will also be fitted with a compression garment to be worn several weeks following your surgery. This garment helps your skin shrink back to better conform to your body. It also reduces postoperative swelling.

Postsurgical Guidelines

Although it may take up to six months to fully heal after surgery, you can usually walk around right after your surgery. Most surgeons advise that you can drive and return to work after about a week. In two weeks, it's fine to engage in some low-intensity exercise. Sexual activity can be resumed in two weeks. After a month, you should be able to engage in more strenuous exercise.

You'll be given a detailed set of other postoperative instructions too, and these should be followed to the letter to avoid complications.

You'll see a noticeable difference in your appearance right after surgery. As swelling goes down, you'll notice more improvement over the course of several weeks. In about three months, the final contour of your reshaped figure will be visible. To prevent unwanted weight gain in the future, you should adhere to a healthy diet and maintain a program of regular exercise.

Risks and Complications of Liposuction

Liposuction, like any surgical procedure, is not without risks and complications. It is critical to understand what they are before you decide to go through with surgery. In addition, be sure to discuss the risks with your surgeon. What follows is a list of potential complications:

- temporary loss of feeling in the skin, due to nerve injury
- excessive bleeding
- dehydration, which can lead to shock
- fluid accumulation that must be drained
- infection
- adverse reactions to the solution used in the procedure
- compromised skin texture, including a worsening of cellulite
- skin discoloration

- body contouring irregularities, due to the removal of too much or too little fat
- thermal injuries to the skin or deeper tissues (a potential complication of UAL because ultrasound generates heat)

Deaths have been associated with liposuction. While I was writing this book, a forty-one-year-old woman in my hometown died from complications related to liposuction. An autopsy showed that a clot of fat made its way into the bloodstream and clogged her lungs. According to a report published in the May 13, 1999, issue of *The New England Journal of Medicine*, several deaths that occurred recently in New York City were linked to the procedure. Three of the patients died from a dramatic decline in blood pressure and heart rate—both of which caused cardiac arrest. The lidocaine used in the solution is known to cause these alarming side effects.

Another patient died from a pulmonary embolism. After liposuction had been performed on her legs, a blood clot formed and traveled to her lungs. The risk of a deadly pulmonary embolism can be minimized by special tests and treatment with anticlotting drugs at home for three to six months after the operation. Nonetheless, there are serious, potentially fatal risks associated with liposuction.

Other Forms of Surgical Body Contouring

Whereas liposuction removes localized fat deposits, a technique known as surgical skin tightening improves the laxity of skin and soft tissues. Often, a combination of the two techniques is used to enhance body contours. Some plastic surgeons believe that surgical skin tightening may help improve cellulite.

Surgical skin tightening is major surgery that involves making incisions in the skin, removing extra skin, pulling skin and muscles together, and stitching them into a new position. This procedure can last anywhere from one hour to five hours. As with any surgery, there are risks associated with surgical skin tightening. You should discuss the potential complications with your plastic surgeon.

A relatively new technique called liposhaving uses a thin tube with a rotating blade to shave off unwanted skin and fat, layer by layer. Thus far, the technique has been used only on faces and necks, but some experts believe that it could be used on thighs. To date though, liposhaving has not been widely used.

How to Find a Qualified Surgeon

The final results of your liposuction depend largely on the skill of the plastic surgeon you select. He or she should be uniquely qualified to perform this surgery and experienced in the procedure. What's more, a surgeon should be an artist of sorts—someone who knows how to recontour your figure according to your own unique body shape.

To find a surgeon with this blend of medical expertise and artistry, here are some important guidelines:

- Research and verify the surgeon's credentials. Your surgeon should be board-certified by the American Society of Plastic and Reconstructive Surgeons (ASPRS), a professional association that represents 97 percent of all board-certified plastic surgeons. Board certification indicates that a surgeon is exceedingly qualified in his or her specialty. You can contact the ASPRS at 444 East Algonquin Road, Arlington Heights, Illinois 60005; 1-847-228-9900. Or access the organization's Web site at www.plasticsurgery.org. On its Web site, you can find information on liposuction and locate a surgeon by name or geographical area.
- Find out how many liposuction procedures a surgeon has performed.
- Ask to see before-and-after photographs of patients, or better yet, talk to former patients.
- Ask to see complication rates—the percentage of patients who have experienced complications and side effects following surgery.

Like many areas of plastic surgery, liposuction is an evolving field, with ongoing improvements in technique and technology. Your challenge is to thoroughly investigate your options—and do so rationally—before jumping into a surgery that carries significant risks.

APPENDIX B

References

A portion of the information in this book comes from medical research reports in both popular and scientific publications, professional textbooks and booklets, books, Internet sources, and computer searches of medical databases of research abstracts.

CHAPTER 1
Toward a Cellulite-Resistant Body

Almasi, M.R. 1994. "The Truth about Cellulite." *Redbook*. June: 46–47.

American Heart Association. 1999. *Heart and Stroke Guide*. Dallas, Texas: American Heart Association.

Berkman, S. 1995. "How to Beat Bloat." *Good Housekeeping*. February: 173–174.

Bernstein, E.F., C.B. Underhill, P.J. Hahn, et al. 1996. "Chronic Sun Exposure Alters Both the Content and Distribution of Dermal Glycosaminoglycans." *British Journal of Dermatology* 135: 255–262.

Biallot, S. 1994. "The Skinny on Cellulite." *Town & Country Monthly*. April: 52–53.

Bouchard, C., G.A. Bray, and V.S. Hubbard. 1990. "Basic and Clinical Aspects of Regional Fat Distribution." *American Journal of Clinical Nutrition* 52: 946–950.

Craig, B. 1989. "Facts About Fat Cells." *Diabetes Forecast* 42: 61–65.

Dancey, E. 1996. *The Cellulite Solution*. New York: St. Martin's Press.

Driedger, S.D. 1996. "The Joy of Being Fat Free: Liposuction Vacuums out Bags and Bulges from Head to Toe." *Maclean's*. July 8: 42.

Editor. 1984. "The Shape of Fatness." *The Lancet* 1: 889.

Editor. 1990. "Goodbye Cellulite?" *The Edell Health Letter*. May: 6.

Editor. 1992. "Calories Aren't Created Equal." *Mayo Clinic Health Letter*. March: 7.

Editor. 1999. "Another Cellulite Remedy." *Harvard Women's Health Watch* 6: 7.

Editor. 1999. "Deaths Related to Liposuction." *The New England Journal of Medicine* 340: 1471–1475.

Evansville Courier. 1998. "Hunger Hormone Believed Found." February 20: A-2.

Gruber, D.M., and J.C. Gruber. 1999. "Gender-Specific Medicine: The New Profile of Gynecology." *Gynecological Endocrinology* 13: 1–6.

Heins, K. 1998. "Estrogen Q and A: Experts Answer Your Questions about the Female Hormone." *Better Homes and Gardens*, October: 144–146.

Illouz, Y.G. 1990. "Study of Subcutaneous Fat." *Aesthetic Plastic Surgery* 14: 165–177.

Kulozik, M., and T. Krieg. 1989. "Changes in Collagen Connective Tissue and Fibroblasts in Aging." *Zeitschrift fur Hautkrankheiten* 64: 1003–1004, 1007–1009.

Lotti, T., I. Ghersetich, C. Grappone, et al. 1990. "Proteoglycans in So-Called Cellulite." *International Journal of Dermatology* 29: 272–274.

Medestea Internazionale, S.R.L., and Rexall Sundown, Inc. 1999. Expert Scientific Paper on Cellasene. May: 13–17.

Nürnberger, F., and G. Müller. 1978. "So-Called Cellulite: An Invented Disease." *Journal of Dermatologic Surgery and Oncology* 4: 221–229.

Raloff, J. 1997. "Getting Older and a Little Rounder?" *Science News*. November 1: 282.

Rosenbaum, M., V. Prieto, J. Hellmer, et al. 1998. "An Exploratory Investigation of the Morphology and Biochemistry of Cellulite." *Plastic and Reconstructive Surgery* 101: 1934–1939.

Ryan, T.J., and S.B. Curri. 1989. "The Structure of Fat." *Clinics in Dermatology* 7: 37–47.

Scherwitz, C., and O. Braun-Falco. 1978. "So-Called Cellulite." *Journal of Dermatologic Surgery and Oncology* 4: 230–234.

Springer, R. 1996. "Liposuction: An Overview." *Plastic Surgical Nursing* 16: 215–224.

Stacey, S. 1997. "Cellulite: The Bottom Line." *Independent on Sunday*. April 20: 4.

Tanada, H., T. Okada, H. Konishi, and T. Tsuji. 1993. "The Effect of Reactive Oxygen Species on the Biosynthesis of Collagen and Glycosaminoglycans in Cultured Human Dermal Fibroblasts." *Archives of Dermatological Research* 285: 352–355.

Tsuji, T., K. Kosaka, and J. Terao. 1989. "Localized Lipodystrophy with Panniculitis: Light and Electron Microscopic Studies." *Journal of Cutaneous Pathology* 16: 359–364.

Whitmore, S.E., and M.A. Levine. 1998. "Risk Factors for Reduced Skin Thickness and Bone Density: Possible Clues Regarding Pathophysiology, Prevention, and Treatment." *Journal of the American Academy of Dermatology* 38: 248–255.

Wright, J.V. 1995. "Retaining Water? Sensitivity to Favorite Foods Could Be Cause." *Health News & Review*. Summer: 2.

CHAPTER 2

Evaluating Your Cellulite

Jensen, M.D. 1992. "Research Techniques for Body Composition Assessment. *Journal of the American Dietetic Association* 92:4 54–459.

Nürnberger, F., and G. Müller. 1978. "So-Called Cellulite: An Invented Disease." *Journal of Dermatologic Surgery and Oncology* 4: 221–229.

Orphanidou, C., L. McCargar, C.L. Birmingham, et al. 1994. "Accuracy of Subcutaneous Fat Measurement: Comparison of Skinfolds, Ultrasound, and Computed Tomography." *Journal of the American Dietetic Association* 94: 855–858.

Potera, C. 1995. "Exercise and Breast Cancer." *The Physician and Sportsmedicine* 23: 37–38.

CHAPTER 3
Cellasene: A Supplement Breakthrough

Beraka, G. 1999. "Revised Interim Report Baseline to Week 8." Unpublished report of Cellasene trial.

Blumenthal, M. 1998. *The Complete German Commission E Monographs: Therapeutic Guide to Herbal Medicines*. American Botanical Council: Austin, Texas.

Duke, J.A. 1997. *The Green Pharmacy*. Emmaus, Pennsylvania: Rodale Press.

Editor. 1999. "Cellulite Researcher Declares Cellasene Works." *Canadian Corporate News*. May 28.

Funston, M. 1999. "Pill to Fight Cellulite on the Market." *The Toronto Star*. March 10.

Gorman, C. 1999. "Cellulite Hype: A Pricey Herbal Pill May Help Eliminate Those Fatty Deposits. But Read This Before You Buy." *Time*. March 22: 115.

Hellmich, N. 1999. "A Big Fat Spat Over a New Way to Fight Cellulite. Doctors Dispute Claims That Cellasene Is a Smooth Solution." *USA Today*. May 25: 13D.

Kalb, C., and K. Springen. 1999. "Fighting Cellulite." *Newsweek*. June 7: 66.

Los Angeles Times. 1999. "Debating a Cellulite 'Cure.'" *Newsday*. April 13.

Medestea Internazionale, S.R.L., and Rexall Sundown, Inc. 1999. Expert Scientific Paper on Cellasene. May.

Taylor, S., and J. Buttriss. 1999. Debate: An Anti-Cellulite Drug, Hailed as a Cure by Its Makers." *Independent on Sunday*. March 14: 5.

TransMedia. 1999. "Cellasene, the Anti-Cellulite Pill that Caused Riots in Australia, Has Reached U.S. Stores Nationwide." News release, March 10.

TransMedia. 1999. "Clinical Studies Showing Effectiveness of Cellasene in Reducing Cellulite Made Public Today." News release, March 25.

CHAPTER 4
Other Cellulite Control Supplements

Blumenthal, M. 1998. *The Complete German Commission E Monographs: Therapeutic Guide to Herbal Medicines*. American Botanical Council: Austin, Texas.

Dolby, V. 1998. "Enzymes: Unlocking the Power of Food." *Better Nutrition*. March: 18.

Duke, J.A. 1997. *The Green Pharmacy*. Emmaus, Pennsylvania: Rodale Press.

Herbst, D. 1999. "Bad Mix." *Natural Health*. September: 100–103, 147.

McCaleb, R. 1993. "Bilberry for Circulatory Health." *Better Nutrition*. June: 54–56.

McCaleb, R. 1994. "Bilberry: Herbal Antioxidant Ripe for the Picking." *Better Nutrition*. November: 56–59.

Schechter, S. 1998. "Power Up with High-Energy Herbs!" *Better Nutrition*. June: 52–55.

CHAPTER 5
Natural Fat Burners

Astrup, A., et al. 1992. "The Effect and Safety of an Ephedrine/Caffeine Compound Compared to Ephedrine, Caffeine and Placebo in Obese Subjects on an Energy Restricted Diet. A double blind trial." *International Journal of Obesity and Related Metabolic Disorders* 16: 269–277.

Cangiano, C., et al. 1992. "Eating Behavior and Adherence to Dietary Prescriptions in Obese Subjects Treated with 5-Hydroxytryptophan." *American Journal of Clinical Nutrition* 56: 863–867.

Clarkson, P.M. 1991. "Nutritional Ergogenic Aids: Chromium, Exercise, and Muscle Mass." *International Journal of Sport Nutrition* 1: 289–293.

Clouatre, D. 1995. *Anti-Fat Nutrients*. San Francisco: Pax Publishing.

Clouatre, D. 1999. "Weight-Loss Aids." *Let's Live*. January: 29–33.

Editor. 1991. "Benefits of Fiber for Dieters." *Nutrition Research Newsletter*. February: 17.

Editor. 1994. "Dietary Fiber Helps Some to Lose Weight." *Better Nutrition*. October: 34.

Editor. 1994. "For Losing Extra Weight, Try Chromium Picolinate." *Better Nutrition*. September: 13.

Editor. 1998. "What You Should Know about Herbal Phen-Fen." *Woman's Day*. February 2: 36.

Federal Drug Administration. 1997. "Warning About Herbal Fenphen." Internet Web address: www.fda.org.

Gormley, J.J. 1997. "A Trio of Health Concerns Is Faced by a Trio of Ayurvedic Herbs." *Better Nutrition*. June: 28.

Gormley, J.J. 1997. "Dietary Chromium Is Safe—and Elemental to Good Health." *Better Nutrition*. March: 18.

Grant, K.E., R.M. Chandler, A.L. Castle, and J.L. Ivy. 1997. "Chromium and Exercise Training: Effect on Obese Women." *Medicine and Science in Sports and Exercise* 29: 992–998.

Kalman, D.S. 1998. "Analyzing the Latest Natural Weight Loss Supplements." *Muscular Development*. July: 96–98, 152–153.

Kalman, D., C. Colker, R. Stark, et al. 1998. "Effect of Pyruvate Supplementation on Body Composition and Mood." *Current Therapeutic Research* 59: 798–802.

Kalsa, K.P. 1996. "Total Herbal Weight Loss." *Let's Live*. December: 62–65.

National Research Council for Health. 1998. Study Report: BioZan.

Nazar, K., et al. 1996. "Phosphate Supplementation Prevents a Decrease of Triidothyronine and Increases Resting Metabolic Rate During Low Energy Diet." *Journal of Physiology and Pharmacology* 47: 373–383.

Passwater, R.A. 1992. *Chromium Picolinate: Breakthrough in Sports Nutrition*. New Canaan, Connecticut: Keats Publishing, Inc.

Phillips, B. 1998. "New Study Supports Fat-Loss Supplement Claims." *Muscle Media*. May: 24–25.

Prokop, D. 1997. *Pyruvate: The Super Strength, Stamina and Weight-Loss Supplement*. Pleasant Grove, Utah: Woodland Publishing.

Roufs, J.B. 1997. *Pyruvate: A Scientific Review and Practical Guide*. Intelligent Nutrition, Inc.

Sahley, B.J., and K. Birkner. 1988. "Stress and Weight Control." *Total Health*, April: 56–59.

Schnirring, L. 1997. "Ephedrine Safety Rules Proposed." *The Physician and Sportsmedicine* 25: 29.

Stanko, R.T., et al. 1986. "Inhibition of Lipid Accumulation and Enhancement of Energy Expenditure by the Addition of Pyruvate and Dihydroxyacetone to a Rat Diet." *Metabolism* 35: 182–186.

Taylor, D.S. 1989. "Amino Acids Aid in Weight Control." *Better Nutrition*. May: 10–12.

Toubro, S., A. Astrup, L. Breum, et al. 1993. "The Acute and Chronic Effects of Ephedrine/Caffeine Mixtures on Energy Expenditure and Glucose Metabolism in Humans." *International Journal of Obesity Related Metabolic Disorders* 17(suppl 3): 73–77.

Trent, L.K., and D. Thielding-Cancel. 1995. "Effects of Chromium Picolinate on Body Composition." *Journal of Sports Medicine and Physical Fitness* 35: 273–280.

CHAPTER 6
Nutritional Support Supplements

American Dietetic Association. 1998. "Position of the American Dietetic Association: Use of Nutritive and Non-Nutritive Sweeteners." *Journal of the American Dietetic Association* 98: 580–588.

Cummings, J.H. 1978. "Nutritional Implications of Dietary Fiber." *American Journal of Clinical Nutrition* 31: 521–529.

Editor. 1999. "Natural Vitamin E Superior to Synthetic." *Nutritional Outlook*. January–February: 56.

Guyton, A.C. 1991. *Textbook of Medical Physiology*. 8th edition. Philadelphia: W.B. Saunders Co.

Hartmann, A., A.M. Niess, M. Grunert-Fuchs, et al. 1995. "Vitamin E Prevents Exercise-Induced DNA Damage." *Mutation Research* April 346: 195–202.

Jenkins, D.J.A., T.M.S. Wolever, V. Vuksan, et al. 1989. "Nibbling Versus Gorging: Metabolic Advantages of Increased Meal Frequency." *The New England Journal of Medicine* 321: 929–931.

Kante, M.M. 1994. "Free Radicals, Exercise, and Antioxidant Supplementation." *International Journal of Sport Nutrition*. 4: 205–220.

Kleiner, S., and M. Greenwood-Robinson. 1996. *High Performance Nutrition*. New York: John Wiley & Sons, Inc.

McBride, J. 1991. "How Sweet It Isn't." *Agricultural News* 39: 20–24.

Pacelli, L.C. 1989. "To Fortify Bones Use Calcium and Exercise." *The Physician and Sportsmedicine* 7: 27–28.

Prince, R.L., M. Smith, I.M. Dick, et al. 1991. "Prevention of Postmenopausal Osteoporosis: A Comparative Study of Exercise, Calcium Supplementation, and Hormone-Replacement Therapy." *New England Journal of Medicine* 325:1189–1195.

Ryttig, K.R., et al. 1989. A Dietary Fibre Supplement and Weight Maintenance after Weight Reduction: A Randomized, Double-Blind, Placebo-Controlled Long-Term Trial." *International Journal of Obesity* 13: 165–171.

CHAPTER 7
Nutritional Cellulite Busters

Clark, N. 1992. "Fluid Facts: What, When, and How Much to Drink." *The Physician and Sportsmedicine* 20: 33–36.

Cummings, J.H. 1978. "Nutritional Implications of Dietary Fiber." *American Journal of Clinical Nutrition* 31: 521–529.

Editor. 1992. "Alcohol and Weight Gain—A Double Whammy." *Medical Update* 16: 4.

Hirsch, J., S.K. Fried, K. Edens, et al. 1989. "The Fat Cell." *Medical Clinics of North America* 73: 83–96.

Judd, P.A., et al. 1981. "The Effect of Rolled Oats on Blood Lipids and Fecal Steroid Excretion in Man." *American Journal of Clinical Nutrition* 34: 2061–2067.

Mazer, E. 1983. "Natural Remedies for Fluid Retention." *Prevention*. December: 106–112.

CHAPTER 9
Downsize Your Thighs

Baker, J. 1994. "Resistance Training Basics: The What, Why and How of a Complete Fitness Program." *American Fitness*. May–June: 26–30.

Brown, R.D., and J.M. Harrison. 1986. "The Effects of a Strength Training Program on the Strength and Self-Concept of Two Female Age Groups." *Research Quarterly for Exercise and Sport* 57: 315–320.

Dupler, T.L., and C. Cortes. 1993. "Effects of a Whole-Body Resistive Training Regimen in the Elderly." *Gerontology* 39: 314–319.

Hilgus, L. 1994. "Lipid in the Gut." *Men's Fitness*. August: 74–75, 110–112.

Olson, A.L., and E. Edelstein. 1968. "Spot Reduction of Subcuta-

229

neous Adipose Tissue." *Research Quarterly for Exercise and Sport* 39: 647–652.

Siplia, S., and H. Suominen. 1995. "Effects of Strength and Endurance Training on Thigh and Leg Mass Muscle and Composition in Elderly Women." *Journal of Applied Physiology* 78: 334–340.

Wang, N., R.S. Hikida, R.S. Staron, and J.A. Simoneau. 1993. "Muscle Fiber Types of Women After Resistance Training—Quantitative Ultrastructure and Enzyme Activity." *Pfluegers Archives of the European Journal of Physiology* 424: 494–502.

CHAPTER 10
Conditioning Your Connective Tissue

Berenburg, C.J. 1993. "In the Final Stretch: Proper Stretching Is the Secret to Safe and Effective Muscle Conditioning." *American Fitness*. March–April: 48–51.

Editor. 1997. "To Stretch or Not to Stretch?" *Tufts University Health & Nutrition Letter*. December: 4–5.

Globus, S. 1997. "Why Stretch?" *Current Health 2*. December: 22–23.

Griffith, K. 1997. "Stretch Out and Relax." *Health*. November–December: 84–89.

Stevens, K. 1998. "A Theoretical Overview of Stretching and Flexibility." *American Fitness*. January–February: 30–36.

CHAPTER 11
Fat-Burning, Body-Toning Aerobics

Bahr, R., and O.M. Sejersted. 1991. "Effect of Intensity of Exercise on Excess Postexercise Oxygen Consumption." *Metabolism:* 836–841.

Editor. 1995. "How to Burn 50 Percent More Calories." *1001 Weight Loss Secrets*. Fall: 4.

Goss, F.L., R.J. Robertson, R.J. Spina, et al. 1989. "Energy Cost of Bench Stepping and Pumping Light Handweights in Trained Subjects." *Research Quarterly for Exercise and Sport* 60: 369–372.

Koszuta, L.E. 1986. "Low-Impact Aerobics: Better Than Traditional Aerobic Dance?" *The Physician and Sportsmedicine* 14: 156–161.

Koszuta, L.E. 1987. "Can Fitness Be Found at the Top of the Stairs?" *The Physician and Sportsmedicine*. 15: 165–169.

Miller, J.F., and B.A. Stamford. 1987. "Intensity and Energy Cost of Weight Walking vs. Running for Men and Women." *Journal of Applied Physiology* 62: 1497–1501.

Olson, A.L., and E. Edelstein. 1968. "Spot Reduction of Subcutaneous Adipose Tissue." *Research Quarterly for Exercise and Sport* 39: 647–652.

CHAPTER 13
Endermologie Against Cellulite

Chang, P., J. Wiseman, T. Jacoby, et al. 1998. "Noninvasive Mechanical Body Contouring (Endermologie): A One-Year Clinical Outcome Study Update." *Aesthetic Plastic Surgery* 22: 145–153.

Editor. 1998. "Beauty: Sayonara Cellulite: Deeper Massage, Better Cosmetic Surgery and Super Nutritional Supplements are the Latest Weapons for Attacking Cellulite." *Flare*. May 1: 64, 66.

Editor. 1998. "Cellulite Meltdown." *Harvard Women's Health Watch* 5: 7.

Editor. 1998. "ESC Medical Commences Body Contouring Clinical trial: SilkLight Device; Company Also Changes Product Name from Silhouette to SilkLight." Business Wire. September.

Ersek, R.A., G.E. Mann, S. Salisbury, et al. 1997. Noninvasive Mechanical Body Contouring: A Preliminary Clinical Outcome Study. *Aesthetic Plastic Surgery* 21: 61–67.

Fodor, B.F. 1997. "Endermologie (LPG): Does It Work?" *Aesthetic Plastic Surgery* 21: 68.

Hellmich, N. 1999. "Massage Therapy Rolls Flab into a Sleeker Look." *USA Today*. May: 13D.

Joseph, J. 1998. "Roll it, Suck it, Cellulite Gone?" ABCNEWS.com. July 1.

Kinney, B.M. 1997. "External Fatty Tissue Massage (the "Endermologie" and "Silhouette" Procedures)." *Plastic and Reconstructive Surgery* 100: 1903–1904.

Librach, P.B. 1998. "Rolling Away the Fat: Massage Technique Says So." *St. Louis Post-Dispatch*. August: G1.

Stacey, S. 1997. "Cellulite: The Bottom Line." *Independent on Sunday*. April 20: 4.

CHAPTER 14
Anticellulite Creams and Lotions

Begoun, P., and K. Jones. 1994. "When It Comes to 'Magic' Thigh Cream, Women Should Not be Fooled." Knight-Ridder/Tribune News Service. May 19.

Belcove, J.L. 1995. "Anti-Cellulite: Boon for Body Sales?" *WWD*. May 12: S6.

Belcove, J.L. 1995. "Clarins Out to Give Body a Lift." *WWD*. November 10: 7.

Bombardelli, E. 1994. "Botanical Derivatives in Function Cosmetics." *Drug & Cosmetic Industry* 154: 44–48.

Dickinson, B.I., and M.L. Gora-Harper. 1996. "Aminophylline for Cellulite Removal." *Annals of Pharmacotherapy* 30: 292–293.

Draelos, Z.D., and K.D. Marenus. 1997. "Cellulite: Etiology and Purported Treatment." *Dermatologic Surgery* 23: 1177–1181.

Editor. 1995. "Cellulite Update." *Cosmopolitan*. October: 282–284.

Editor. 1995. "Elancyl's New Challenge in Battle for Bodycare." *Cosmetics International*. February 25: 1–2.

Editor. 1997. "Downsize Your Thighs." *Good Housekeeping*. May: 69–71.

Editor. 1998. "Beauty: Sayonara Cellulite: Deeper Massage, Better Cosmetic Surgery and Super Nutritional Supplements Are the Latest Weapons for Attacking Cellulite." *Flare*. May 1: 64, 66.

Greenfield, D. 1994. "The Bottom Line on Thigh Creams." *Newsday*. April 7.

Greenway, F.L., and G.A. Bray. 1987. "Regional Fat Loss from the Thigh in Obese Women after Adrenergic Modulation." *Clinical Therapeutics* 9: 663–669.

Greenway, F.L., G.A. Bray, and D. Heber. 1995. "Topical Fat Reduction." *Obesity Research* 3: 561S–568S.

Griffin, K. 1994. "A Thigh-Slimming Cream That Works." *Health* March–April: 36–37.

Gurevitch, R. 1998. "The Market Goes Holistic." *WWD*. July 10: 17S.

Hoppe, U., et al. 1999. "Coenzyme Q10, a Cutaneous Antioxidant and Energizer." *Biofactors* 9: 371–378.

Kaats, G.R., D. Pullin, P.L. Tschirhart, et al. "Topical Application of an Aminophylline Thigh Cream: Effect on Blood Chemistries." *Drug & Cosmetic Industry* 155: 28–32.

Kim, S.J., J.H. Park, D.H. Kim, et al. 1998. "Increased In Vivo Collagen Synthesis and In Vitro Cell Proliferative Effect of Glycolic Acid." *Dermatologic Surgery* 24: 1054–1058.

Lieberman, J., and L. McRee. 1998. "The Buck Starts Here." *ABC Good Morning America*. February 16.

Lower, E. 1997. "Smoothing Over the Problem." *Soap Perfumery & Cosmetics*. April 1: 55.

Marks, B.L., L.M. Katz, J.E. Haky, et al. 1999. "Spectral Analysis of Heart Rate Variability and Pulmonary Response to Topical Applications of 2% Aminophylline-Based Cream." *International Journal of Obesity and Related Metabolic Disorders* 23: 108–202.

Naiman, S. 1999. "A Bumpy Blight on the Bumscape: Women Obsessed with Cellulite, Doctors Say." *Toronto Sun*. January 25: 45.

Rae, S. 1991. "Retin-A: Acne Remedy or Wrinkle Reducer?" *Modern Maturity*. December–January: 76.

Rae, S. 1991. "Wrapping the Human Package: Your Skin Holds You Together So Treat It with Respect." *Modern Maturity*. June–July: 72–76.

Ranard, A. 1989. "Between the Lines." *Health*. October: 66–69.

Smith, W.P. 1996. "Epidermal and Dermal Effects of Topical Lactic Acid." *Journal of the American Academy of Dermatology* 35: 388–391.

Stenson, J. 1999. "Thigh Creams Don't Melt Fat Away, After All." MSNBC.com. July 3.

Turnis, J. 1994. "New Creams Smooth Cellulite, but Thin Thighs from Bottle Are Several Years Away." Knight-Ridder/Tribune News Service. April 1.

Williams, C. 1997. "Cream Crackers." *Independent on Sunday*. June 1: 9.

Young, R.K. 1988. "Cellulite: Fact or Fiction." *American Fitness*. April: 28–29.

APPENDIX A
Should You Consider Liposuction?

Ablaza, V.J., M.R. Jone, M.K. Gingrass, et al. 1998. "Ultrasound Assisted Lipoplasty." *Plastic Surgical Nursing* 18: 13–25.

Adamo, C., M. Mazzocchi, A. Rossi, et al. 1997. "Ultrasonic Liposculpturing: Extrapolations from the Analysis of In Vivo Sonicated Adipose Tissue." *Plastic and Reconstructive Surgery* 100: 220–226.

American Academy of Dermatology. 1998. "Ultrasonic Liposuction: Reinventing the Wheel?" Press release. February 28.

American Society of Plastic and Reconstructive Surgeons. 1999. Internet Web site: www.plasticsurgery.org.

Editor. 1996. "Bye-Bye Thighs." *Industry Week*. February 5: 19.

Editor. 1997. "Sound Waves to Break Up Fat." *USA Today Magazine*. October: 15–16.

Hirsch, J., S.K. Fried, K. Edens, et al. 1989. "The Fat Cell." *Medical Clinics of North America* 73: 83–96.

Igra, H., and N.M. Satur. 1997. "Tumescent Liposuction versus Internal Ultrasonic-Assisted Tumescent Liposuction: A Side-by-Side comparison." *Dermatologic Surgery* 23: 1213–1218.

Lockwood, T. 1996. "The Role of Excisional Lifting in Body Contouring Surgery." *Clinics in Plastic Surgery* 23: 695–712.

Springer, R. 1996. "Liposuction: An Overview." *Plastic Surgical Nursing* 16: 215–224.

Zimmer, J. 1998. "Body Work." *Essence*. August: 17–21.

INDEX

Maggie Greenwood-Robinson, Ph.D.

Maggie Greenwood-Robinson, Ph.D. is one of the country's top health and medical authors. She is the author of *Kava: The Ultimate Guide to Nature's Anti-Stress Herb*, *Hair Savers for Women: A Complete Guide to Treating and Preventing Hair Loss*, *Natural Weight Loss Miracles*, and *21 Days to Better Fitness;* and the co-author of nine other fitness books, including the national best-seller *Lean Bodies*, *Lean Bodies Total Fitness*, *High Performance Nutrition*, *Power Eating*, and *50 Workout Secrets*.

Her articles have appeared in *Let's Live* magazine, *Great Life*, *Christian Single* magazine, *Women's Sports and Fitness*, *Working Woman*, *Muscle and Fitness*, *Female Bodybuilding and Fitness*, and many other publications. She currently writes "The Natural Dieter" column for *Let's Live*.

Maggie is a member of the Advisory Board of *Physical Magazine*. In addition, she has taught bodyshaping classes at the University of Southern Indiana. Maggie has a doctorate in nutritional counseling and is a certified nutritional consultant.